Lecture Notes in Medical Diagnosis and Treatment

CYR61: Angiogenic Marker in Fracture Healing and its Clinical Implications

Lecture Notes in Medical Diagnosis and Treatment

CYR61: Angiogenic Marker in Fracture Healing and its Clinical Implications

Ajai Singh

Sabir Ali

Published by iConcept Press Limited

Contents

Preface

The fracture healing is a postnatal regenerative process that recapitulates many events of embryonic skeletal development. Although fracture repair usually have the potential to regain its pre-injury cellular composition, structure and biomechanical function, about 10% of fractures will not heal normally. Long bone fractures are the most common traumatic injuries to the human beings, in which tibial bones are the most common one.

Presently there is no standard criteria exist for diagnosing fracture impaired union early. Till date clinico-radiological examination are most commonly used for assessment of fracture healing progression. But due to lack of objectivity the assessment of fracture healing varies among orthopaedic surgeons. This variability can be problematic in both clinical and orthopaedic trauma research settings. Also inability to predict impaired healing early also charges extra cost, morbidity, long time hospitalization to the patients.

An understanding of risk factors for impaired healing and of diagnostic tests used to assess fracture healing outcomes early can facilitate a systematic approach to provide a better assessment and management of fractures. Therefore to overcome the current limitations of clinico-radiological assesment of fracture healing, over the past few decades, scientists and clinicians have been trying to exploring the use of different biomarkers that may reflect the bone turnover process and might be used as a marker to predict the healing impairment early. Angiogenesis plays a crucial role during intramembranous bone formation and endochondral ossification. Cysteine Rich Angiogenic Inducer 61 (CYR61) is one of the marker which was express during angiogenesis as well as bone remodeling process.

CYR61: Angiogenic Marker in Fracture Healing and its Clinical Implications provides current information regarding the biology of fracture repair, reviews the importance of angiogenesis during fracture repair and explores one of the angiogenic biomarker, the CYR61 in predicting the healing outcome early. The authors have thoughtfully and skillfully provided current knowledge in this exciting area. This book should be of value to those in training, clinicians, and basic scientists interested in biology of biomarkers in relation to repair of the musculoskeletal system.

Acknowledgement

I would like to express my gratitude to Department of Biochemistry, King George's Medical University, Lucknow, Uttar Pradesh, India for their kind support. We also acknowledge the financial support provided by Indian Council of Medical Research, New Delhi, India, to successfully conduct the research. Last but not least we also express our gratitude to the Editor-in Chief for their kind support in bringing out this book.

Ajai Singh
Professor
Department of Orthopaedic Surgery
King George's Medical University
Lucknow

Sabir Ali
PhD Scholar
Department of Orthopaedic Surgery
King George's Medical University
Lucknow

1

Introduction

Fractures are common orthopaedic problem and it occurs most in long bones. Amongst all long bones, shaft of tibia is one of the commonest bones that are prone to fractures. Such fractures have relatively higher incidence of impaired healing as the fracture site has lesser soft tissue coverage, because of subcutaneous bone on anterior aspect (Reed et al., 2008; Patel et al., 2009). The mentioned reasons account for a high rate of tibial non-unions amounting to 2-10% of all tibial fractures which leads to significant patient morbidity (Marsh D, 1999; Praemer et al., 1992; Sarmiento et al., 2012). Some authors define non-union as the cessation of all reparative healing processes without bone union till 6 months from the time of fracture (Hernigou et al., 2005). The term "Delayed Union" is used when fracture union has not been achieved and a considerable period of time has elapsed since the initial injury but bone regenerative process of fracture healing is still evident. A number of risk factors that contribute to the development of fracture leading to non-union nature have been identified over the years. These include local and systemic factors that could be related to the fracture personality as a result of the initial insult, the treatment provided or the patient's specific characteristics and co-morbidities (Day et al., 2001; Giannoudis et al., 2005; Calori et al., 2007). Non-union fracture is a dreaded complication with devastating outcomes for the patients. Most of the time, a complex and expensive treatment are required involving multiple surgical procedures, pain, morbidity, prolonged hospital stay and functional and psychosocial disability (Ashman et al., 2013; Giannoudis et al., 2007). The implementation of treatment protocols for such clinical situation can be complex and long-lasting (Calori et al., 2011). Moreover, the consequent socio-economic burden on patients & then families should not be underestimated (Giannoudis et al., 2007). Ability in prompt identification of patients who are at high risk of non-union will enable early appropriate targeted treatment intervention leading to a successful outcome (Axelrad et al., 2011; Gelalis et al., 2012). Such approach would benefit not only the patient's wellbeing but also the health care system in terms of the cost implications associated with long lasting treatment interventions and prolonged hospital stay.

Fracture healing is a normal physiological process. This is one of the most complex physiological processes aiming to the repair of the fractured bone without the formation of scar tissue (Giannoudis et al., 2011; Mckibbin B, 1978). Healing is continuous process to achieve union (Davis et al. 2004). Therefore, healing should be measured. There are no methods as yet, to measure rates of these processes and quantify the healing process. According to Wade et al. (2001) a valid measurement for union should be measurable at each point of time during the union process. Thus, the values obtained by measurement should be on a continuous numeric scale. Currently, clinical and radiological methods are most common tools to assess the healing of fractures. According to Hammer et al. (1985) the probability of correct radiological evaluation of fractures union of tibia has been shown to be only about 50%. A study on radiological evaluation of the stage of union in fractures of tibia found that the radiographic assessment is not a most suitable method to assess fracture healing (McCloskey et al. 1993). According to Marsh et al. (1998) none of the measures of union will help early detection of problems related with healing. The clinico-radiological method will not help the clinician to identify delayed and non-unions in anticipation at the time of start of treatment. In such case, the patient had to suffer for a long period of time.

Moreover, treating doctors have conventionally relied on clinical and radiological assessment to remove plasters but these methods lack objectivity and hence are not a reliable to compare "time to union" in different treatment methods. Hence, there is a need to develop an accurate, reliable, reproducible and cost-effective method to measure fracture healing objectively. Apart from being accurate, precise, reliable and cost-effective, the method should be acceptable to the patients as well as the treating doctors.

Cox et al. (2010) observed that the biochemical markers of bone-turnover have been used to complement the radiological assessment of patients with metabolic bone disease. Since they are derived from both cortical and trabecular bones, they reflect the metabolic activity of the entire skeleton rather than that of individual cells or the process of mineralization. Quantitative changes in skeletal-turnover can be assessed easily and non-invasively by the analyzing the of bone-turnover markers.

Angiogenesis is the process of formation of new blood vessels from pre-existing ones. After fracture it is stimulated to maintain oxygen homeostasis, supply of nutrients, and removal of the waste products as well as provide cells and biological mediators. Angiogenesis plays a crucial role during intramembranous bone formation and endochondral ossification (Harper and Klagsbrun, 1999). An adequate blood supply to the fracture is a prerequisite for the reconstitution of bone tissue, whereas insufficient blood supply is likely to result in impaired bone healing (Hausman et al., 2001).

The Cysteine Rich Angiogenic Inducer 61 (CYR61) gene is key indicative molecule involved in angiogenesis. In previous studies, it was found that the CYR61 is an extracellular signaling molecule in human bone (Babic et al., 1998; Kolesnikova anf Lau, 1998; Lechner et al., 2000). According to O'Brien and Lau, (1992) CYR61 acts as a novel player in chondrogenesis. They also suggested that CYR61 may be important for the normal growth, differentiation, or morphogenesis of the cartilaginous skeleton of the embryo (O'Brien and Lau, 1992). Furthermore Hadjiargyrou et al. (2000) and Jasmin et al. (2005) primarily identified CYR61 to be up-regulated during fracture healing. They suggested that CYR61 plays a vital role in cartilage and bone formation and may act as an important regulator of fracture healing.

Due to rapid accumulation of new knowledge of bone matrix physiology and biochemistry, attempts have been made to use them in the interpretation and characterization of various stages of the healing of fractures. Early knowledge of the individual progress of a fracture could help to avoid delayed or nonunion by enabling modification of the host's biological response. The level of biomarkers varies throughout the course of fracture repair as their rates of change are dependent on the size of the fracture and the time it will take to heal.

The present study indents to angiogenic marker (CYR61) responsible for healing of fractures at the time of start of the treatment procedure. With help of this marker, prognosis of a fracture case could be predicted and a suitable intervention could be planned at appropriate time. This would minimize suffering of the patient. In this we planned to quantify CYR61 expression (mRNA and protein) in whole blood at the early phase of healing in patients with simple diaphyseal tibial fracture. The clinico-radiological progression could be compared with biochemical expression (at different time periods; which may give fruitful information regarding their expressions at different stage of early healing. This may give clinicians an optimum, sensitive and specific tool for the diagnosis of impaired union early.

2

Physiology of Fracture Healing

2.1   Introduction

Fracture shaft of tibia is a common but unexpected trauma in adults which results in painful and prolonged recovery and is often associated with complications (Alt et al., 2009; Hak et al., 2011). According to U.S. National Center for Health Statistics, approximately 4,92,000 new cases of fractures of tibia, fibula, and ankle are reported annually (Praemer et al., 1992). Annual incidence of fracture tibia and fibula results in 77,000 hospitalizations, making-up to a total of 569,000 hospital days and 825,000 physician office visits (Miller et al., 2007). According to U.S. Agency for Healthcare Research and Quality (AHRQ), 151,966 hospital discharges were reported in 2007 for which tibia/fibula fractures were responsible for a principal procedure (AHQR Report, 2007). Outcome of tibial fractures depend on treatment options which vary on the basis of injury type, its severity and associated complications (Bhandari et al., 2001; Johnson et al. 2008). Non-union or delayed union is a common late complication of fracture shaft of tibia (Bhandari et al., 2001; Minoo et al., 2011). For tibial non-union there is no specific definition, but according to some authors tibial non-union is defined as a fracture that would not unite without additional surgical or non-surgical intervention in 6–9 months period (Minoo et al., 2011), while others preferred to wait for six month before performing surgeries to faultless non-unions (Bhandari et al., 2008). An expectant management, followed by non-invasive therapies such as low-intensity pulsed ultrasound or vibration is a conventional approach to delayed unions (Kasturi et al., 2011; Martinez et al., 2011; Nolte et al., 2001). If healing fails within a clinically reasonable time period, i.e., 6–9 months, a second surgical intervention becomes mandatory to stabilize the fracture (Minoo et al., 2011; Bhandari et al., 2008). Further, in secondary therapies, different adjuvants used during the surgery, may also improve the bony healing process, but they are costly or associated with morbidity. Therefore, tibial fractures cause substantial morbidity, healthcare use, and extra costs. An effective screening for risk factors leading to nonunion and evaluation of biomarkers for early detection of nonunion in tibial or any fracture healing is expected to decrease the morbidity, burden on healthcare resource and cost incurred on treatment.

2.2 Tibial Shaft Fracture Healing

There are two types of bone-cortical and cancellous which complement the supporting, protective, and mechanical functions of the skeleton. The cortical bone constructs the shafts of the long bones (appendicular skeleton) that are presumed to be approximately 80% of the skeletal mass (Nelson B. Watts, 1999). The spongy (cancellous or trabecular bone) bone has a lacy or honey-combed pattern. It provides a reservoir for minerals, with a large surface area and is the best site for bone forming cells. It comprises the inner parts of the bones of the vertebrae, pelvis and end of long bones of extremities.

On contrary to soft tissue healing that leads to scar formation, bone is amongst one of the few tissues which can heal without forming a fibrous scar and this is unique to it. Likewise, fracture healing recapitulates bone development process and can be considered as a form of tissue regeneration (Marsell et al., 2010). The ultimate result of fracture healing is the regeneration of the anatomy of the bone with proper functioning.

Fracture healing can be distinguished into two main categories: (1) Primary (direct, cortical) bone healing, and (2) Secondary (indirect, spontaneous) bone healing. Both healing processes are complex in nature. This process includes coordination of sequence of various biological events.

2.2.1   Primary Bone Healing

The primary (Direct) bone healing generally does not take place in the process of natural fracture healing. It needs a rigid stabilization with or without compression of the bone ends. In comparison to secondary bone healing, this rigid stabilization inhibits the formation of a callus in either cancellous or cortical bone (Allgower et al., 1979; Muller et al., 1965; Perren et al., 1979; 1987; 1989). Because most fractures occurring worldwide are either untreated or treated in a way that results in some degree of motion (sling or cast immobilization, external or intramedullary fixation), primary healing is rare (Thomas et al., 1998). Though some have considered this type of healing to be a goal of fracture repair, yet in many ways it is not shown to be advantageous over secondary bone healing (Rahn et al., 1971; Schenk el al., 1963). The intermediate stages are weak, do not occur in an anaerobic environment (Madison et al.,1993). Primary bone healing can be divided further into gap healing and contact healing. Both of these are able to achieve bone union without external callus formation and any fibrous tissue or cartilage formation within the fracture gap.

2.2.1.1   Gap Healing

Gap healing generally occurs in two stages: initially by bone filling followed by the remodelling process. The width of the gap is first filled by direct bone formation. In the process of gap healing, the initial scaffold of the woven bone is laid down, followed by the formation of parallel-fibered and/or lamellar bone as support (Schenk et al., 1967). The orientation of the new bone formed at the initial stage is transverse to the original lamellar bone orientation. After several weeks, second stage of gap healing initiates, in which the longitudinal haversian remodelling reconstructs the necrotic fracture ends and the newly formed bone is replaced with osteons having original orientation (DeLacure et al., 1994). At the end of normal gap healing, the bone structure is return to same as it was before the fracture.

2.2.1.2   Contact Healing

Contact healing usually occurs when the bone fragments are in direct appo-sition and the osteons grow across the fracture site. Contrary to gap healing, in which transverse bone formation occurs between fracture ends, in contact healing the growth is parallel to the long axis of the bone without being pre-ceded by the process of transverse bone formation between fracture ends (Perren et al., 1979; Schenk et al., 1967). Further, the osteoclasts on one side of the fracture undergo a resorptive response, forming cutting cones which allows the penetration of capillary loops and formation of new haversian systems. The blood vessels are accompanied by endothelial cells and oste-oprogenitor cells for osteoblasts that lead to the production of osteons across the fracture line (Thomas et al., 1998). The result of normal contact healing will also eventually lead to regeneration of the normal bone architecture.

2.2.2   Secondary Bone Healing

The commonest type of bone healing is secondary (Indirect) fracture healing. It generally takes place in the absence of rigid fixation of the fracture site. On the contrary, it is enhanced by micro-motion and weight-bearing. However, too much motion and/or load leads to delayed healing or even non-union (Green et al.,2005). Indirect bone healing typically occurs in non-operative fracture treatment and in certain operative treatments in which some motion occurs at the fracture site such as intramedullary nailing, external fixation, or internal fixation of complicated comminuted fractures (Pape et al.,2002; Perren et al., 2002).

Although, many studies reports the entire process of fracture healing in three to five phases (Cruess et al., 1975; Madison et al., 1993; Frost et al., 1989; McKibbin et al., 1978; Thomas et al., 1998; Marsh et al., 1999), the fracture healing mainly comprises of three phases: an inflammatory phase; a reparative phase (involves intramembranous ossification, chondrogenesis, and endochondral ossification) and a remodelling phase (Cruess et al. 1975; Bolander et al.,1992). Since healing is a complex phenomenon, it is crucial to note that these three phases overlap each another during the healing process. These phases are described as follows:

Stage of Bone Healing

Reactive phase	Reparative phase	Remodeling phase
Fracture and inflammatory phase	Cartilage callus formation	Remodeling to original bone contour
Granulation tissue formation	Lamellar bone deposition	

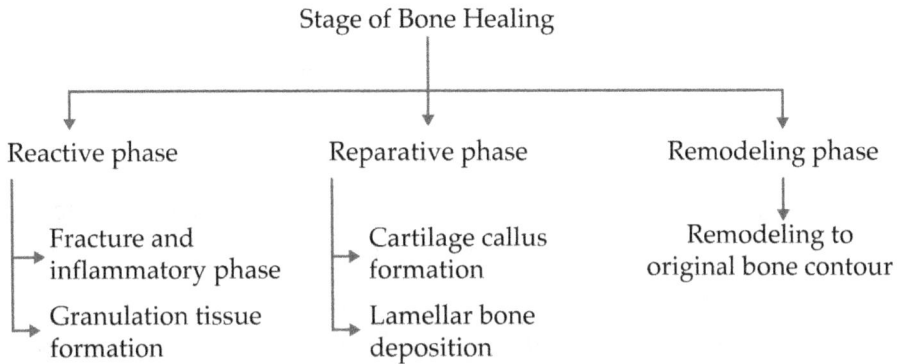

Figure 2.1: Illustrating four major phases of fracture healing.

2.2.2.1   Inflammatory Phase

Fracture damages the bone cells, blood vessels and bone matrix, as well as injury to the surrounding soft tissues (Buckwalter et al., 1996). An instant anti-inflammatory response is generated, which maximizes in 48 hours and then entirely vanishes by 1 week after fracture. Vascular endothelial damage activates the complement cascade, platelet aggregation and degranulation, and release of its α-granule contents at the fracture site. Angiogenesis is activated by polymorphonuclear leukocytes (PMNs), tissue macrophages, lymphocytes and blood monocytes (Glowacki et al., 1998). Initially, the conditions at fracture site are generally hypoxic and acidic, which is ideal for the PMNs activities and tissue macrophages (Hollinger et al., 1996). Hematoma is gathered in medullary canal within the fracture ends and under the elevated periosteum and muscles(Madison et al., 1993; Buckwalter et al., 1996; Grundnes et al.,1993a; Grundnes et al.,1993b). Thus, produced hematoma followed by the trauma, constitutes cells from both peripheral and intramedullary blood, also the bone marrow cells (Gerstenfeld et al., 2003). Hematoma is reported as a source of signalling molecules to trigger vital cellular events during fracture healing (Bolander et al., 1992). The result leads the hematoma to coagulate within and around the fracture ends and inside the medulla preparing a template for development of callus (Gerstenfeld et al., 2003).

2.2.2.2   Reparative Phase

The reparative phase eventuates within the first few days prior to the inflammatory phase, subsides and resides for many weeks. In this phase, the formation of a reparative callus tissue within and nearby the fracture site will eventually be replaced by bone. The function of the callus is to provide strength and mechanical stability at the fracture site by bracing it. Osteocytes found at the fracture ends become deficient in nutrients and die that is noticed by the presence of empty lacunae extending for some distance from the fracture (McKibbin et al., 1978). The damaged periosteum, marrow and other surrounding soft tissues may also contribute to necrotic tissue at the fracture site (Madison et al.,1993).The pluripotent mesenchymalcells start forming other cells like fibroblasts, chondroblasts, and osteoblasts. Through-out this phase, the callus can comprise of fibrous connective tissue, blood vessels, cartilage, woven bone, and osteoid. When the repair progresses, the pH slowly becomes neutral and then slightly alkaline, that is suitable for alkaline phosphatase activity and its role in the mineralization of the callus (Buckwalter et al., 1996). It is already revealed that the first bone formed is from the cells in the cambium layer of the periosteum (Tonna et al., 1963). The rate of repair may vary depending on the location of fracture in bone, the amount of soft tissue damage and mechanical stability at the fracture site (Buckwalter et al., 1996). A closer look at the reparative phase focuses on intramembranous ossification, chondrogenesis, and endochondral ossifycat-ion.

Intramembranous ossification starts between first few days of fracture, but the proliferative activities appear to stop within 2 week after the fracture. Histological facts first show the osteoblast activity in the woven bone that opposed to the cortex within a few mill meters from the fracture site (Thomas et al. 1998). Bone formation starts at this site with the differentiation from osteoblasts. It occurs directly from precursor cells and does not involve formation of cartilage as an intermediate step. This type of bone formation occurring in the external callus is often referred to as the hard callus (Bolander et al., 1992).

Due to low oxygen stress, chondrogenesis takes place in the callus periphery simultaneously with intramembranous ossification. (McKibbin et al., 1978). In granulation tissue at the fracture site, undifferentiated or mesenchymal cells formed the periosteum and neighbouring external soft tissues (Thomas et al., 1998). These cells grow further and start to appear like cartilage and begin to synthesize an avascular basophilic matrix in the same way as it is seen in the proliferating zone of the growth plate. This region of fibrous tissue and new cartilage is referred to as the soft callus. The soft callus would ultimately replace all fibrous tissue (Bolander et al., 1992).

By the middle of the second week of fracture healing process, there is ample amount of cartilage overlying at the fracture area and calcification begins by the process of endochondral ossification (Thomas et al., 1998). This process is much like the one seen in the growth plate. Hypertrophic chondrocytes initially secrete neutral proteoglycanases which degrades glycosaminoglycans, because of high levels of glycosaminoglycans inhibit mineralization (Einhorn et al., 1989). Subsequently, these cells followed by osteoblasts, release membrane-derived vesicles which contain calcium phosphate complexes into the matrix (Brighton et al., 1986). These membrane derived vescicles also carry neutral proteases and alkaline phosphatase enzymes that degrade the proteoglycan-rich matrix and hydrolyze high-energy phosphate esters in order to provide phosphate ions for precipitation with calcium (Buckwalter et al., 1996). While the mineralization process progresses, the callus calcification becomes more rigid and the fracture site is considered to be internally stabilized (Madison et al., 1993). Capillaries from adjacent bone tissue invades the calcified cartilage and results in elevation of the oxygen tension. This is followed by invasion of osteoblasts which forms primary spongiosa involving both cartilage and woven bone (Bolander et al., 1992). Eventually the callus is composed of just-woven bone, which joins the two fracture ends, and the remodelling process begins at this point.

2.2.2.3   Remodeling Phase

Bone remodeling is also called bone turnover. It is an essential part of bone health. Due to daily activities, bone sustains micro-fractures and fatigue.

Such damage must be repaired to ensure bone strength. Without remodeling, the skeleton would eventually collapse. Remodeling is regulated by both local and systemic factors. These factors include electrical and mechanical forces, hormones (e.g., parathyroid hormone, thyroid hormone, vitamin D and its metabolites, estrogen, androgens, cortisol, calcitonin, and growth hormone), growth factors (e.g., insulin-like growth factor 1 (IGF-1) and transforming growth factor), and cytokines (e.g., interleukins 1 and 6).

Remodeling takes place only on the surface of bone and in closely co-ordinated local packets. The cells involved in a particular remodeling event are referred to as a basic multicellular unit or bone metabolic unit (BMU). In a typical remodeling cycle, resorption takes 7–10 days, whereas formation requires 2–3 months. Approximately 10% of total bone is replaced each year. Remodeling occurs exclusively on bone surfaces. Cancellous bone makes up 20% of the skeletal mass and 80% of the surface area. Therefore, cancellous bone is metabolically more active and more rapidly remodeled than cortical bone. Approximately 25% of cancellous bone is renewed each year as compared to 3% of cortical bone (Nelson B. Watts, 1999).

The bone remodeling process is generally referred as "Coupled". Coupling means the bone formation is linked to bone resorption and bone formation must be preceded by bone resorption. There are rare exceptions to the "Coupling" theory. Coupling should not be confused with balance. Balance means that the amount of bone that is removed is entirely replaced with new bone. However, after the age of 35–40, each time a remodeling cycle is completed there is a net loss of bone because the amount of bone formed is less than the amount removed by resorption. Deficiency of estrogen and other abnormalities of skeletal regulation greatly increase the rate of remodeling and accentuate this imbalance.

In a normal bone, the biomechanical properties cannot be completely restored by the hard callus. However, it is a rigid structure which provides biomechanical stability. To attain this property, the fracture healing cascade inculcates a second resorptive phase with hard callus reconstructed into a lamellar bone structure with medullar cavity in the center (Gerstenfeld et al., 2003). Remodelling phase is the last stage of fracture healing which starts with the replacement of woven bone by lamellar bone and excess callus is resorbed (Buckwalter et al. 1996; Hollinger et al., 1996). Although the process begins as early as 3–4 weeks in animal and human models, the remodeling may take years to complete and to get an entirely regenerated bone structure (Wendeberg et al., 1961). In addition to replacement of all constructed bone, remodelling of fracture repair comprises of osteoclasticresorption of poorly located trabeculae and development of new bone along the lines of stress (Frost et al., 1989). The process of the remodelling and modelling continues till the optimal stability is achieved, whereas the bone cortex is almost similar to the architecture it had before the occurrence of fracture (Madison et al.,1993).

3

Cysteine-Rich Angiogenic Inducer 61 in Fracture Healing

3.1 Introduction

In humans, the cysteine-rich angiogenic inducer 61 gene encodes a matricellular protein classified as CCN family member 1 (CCN1) also known as CYR61 protein (Jay et al., 1997; Lau et al., 2011; Jun et al., 2011). CYR61 is capable of regulating a broad range of cellular activities including cell adhesion, migration, proliferation, differentiation, apoptosis, and senescence through interaction with cell surface integrin receptors and heparin sulfate proteoglycans. While in embryonic development, CYR61 is vital for cardiac septal morphogenesis, blood vessel formation in placenta, and vascular integrity. In adulthood, CYR61 plays an important role in inflammation and tissue repair and is associated with diseases related to chronic inflammation like rheumatoid arthritis, atherosclerosis, diabetes-related nephropathy and retinopathy, and many different forms of cancers. CYR61 was first identified as a protein encoded by a serum-inducible gene in mouse fibroblasts (Lau et al., 2011). Other highly conserved homologs were later identified to comprise the CCN protein family (CCN intercellular signaling protein) (Leask et al., 2006; Holbourn et al., 2008; Chen et al., 2009). The CCN acronym is derived from the first three members of the family identified, namely CYR61 (CCN1), CTGF (connective tissue growth factor, or CCN2), and NOV (nephroblastoma overexpressed, or CCN3). These proteins, along with WISP1 (CCN4), WISP2 (CCN5), and WISP3 (CCN6) comprise the six members of the family in vertebrates and have been renamed CCN1-6 in order of their discovery by international consensus (Brigstock et al., 2003a). CCN proteins works as matricellular proteins, which are extracellular matrix proteins that play regulatory roles, especially in context of wound repair (Bornstein et al., 2002).

The human cysteine-rich protein 61 (hCYR61) regulated by 1alpha, 25-dihydroxyvitamin D(3) (1,25-(OH)(2)D(3)) belongs to the growing CCN (CYR61/CTGF/NOV) family of immediate early genes which modulate cell growth and differentiation. The hCYR61 acts as a growth factors in fetal human osteoblasts (hFOB cells), identified as an extracellular matrix-associated protein that modulates basic fibroblast growth factor signaling, angiogenesis, and binds to integrin alpha(v)beta(3). The hCYR61 is secreted in primary osteoblasts and hFOB cells. As the N-terminal 34 amino acids of hCYR61, a truncated CYR61-GFP fusion protein provides a sufficient Golgi targeting sequence. Jointly with the immediate early regulation of CYR61 mRNA by 1,25-(OH)(2)D(3), suggest that CYR61 might function as an extracellular signaling molecule in human bone (Lechner et al, 2000).

3.2   Role of Cysteine-Rich Angiogenic Inducer 61 in Fracture Healing

Bone healing is an effective process, but delayed union and non-union are challenging problems which may occur following certain fractures or osteotomies. In such an abnormal healing situation, certain healing processes such as failure of blood supply and factors regulating these processes may be deficient. There is limited literature available on the patho-physiology of healing leading to delayed/non-union.

Angiogenesis, the formation of new blood vessels from pre-existing ones, is stimulated after fracture to maintain oxygen homeostasis, deliver nutrients, remove waste products, and provide cells and biological media-tors. Additionally, angiogenesis plays a crucial role during intramembra-nous bone formation and endochondral ossification (Harper et al., 1999) (Figure 3.1). It was revealed recently that bone marrow derived endothelial progenitor cells are recruited into fracture sites and contribute to local blood vessel formation that is consistent with postnatal vasculogenesis (Matsu-moto et al., 2008).

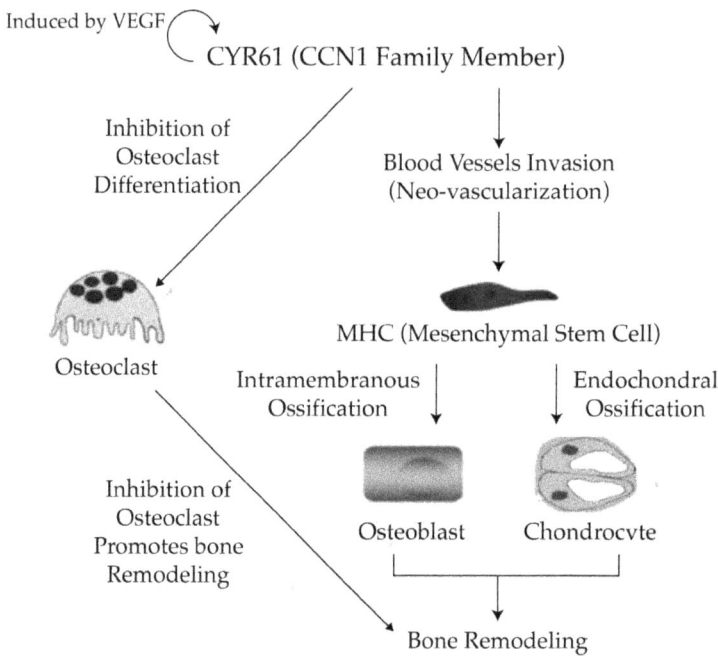

Figure 3.1: The CYR61 protein is expressed in MSCs, osteoblast and chondrocyte via process of blood vessels invasion (neo-vasculariza-tion). The differentiation capacity of the bone is improved by CYR61 expression in osteoblasts. On the other hand osteoclasts are inhibited by CYR61. Therefore, CYR61 shows a crucial role in bone remodeling process.

An adequate blood supply to the fracture is a prerequisite for the re-constitution of bone tissue. Insufficient blood supply is likely to result in de-layed/non-union (Hausman et al., 2001). However, there has been little investigation regarding regulation of blood vessel formation in abnormal bone healing. The formation of new blood vessels is a prerequisite for bone healing, especially for the replacement of cartilage by bone (Marsh et al., 1999). Angiogenesis is a complex process and is regulated by many factors. The cysteine-rich protein 61 (CYR61, CCN1) is an extracellular matrix-associated angiogenic regulator of the CYR61/connective tissue growth factor (CTGF)/nephroblastoma over expressed (CCN) protein family (Brigstock et al., 2003b; O'Brien et al., 1990; Perbal et al., 2004; Yang et al., 1991) consisting of matricellular signaling molecules (Bornstein et al., 2002). CYR61 is basically recognized as the product of an immediate-early gene that is transcriptionally activated by serum and serum growth factors in fibroblasts (O'Brien et al., 1990). CYR61 supports cell adhesion, stimulates endothelial cell migration, enhances growth factor-induced cell proliferation in culture (Kireeva et al., 1996) and induces angiogenesis in vivo (Babic et al., 1998; Fataccioli et al., 2002). Furthermore, a direct proliferative action of CYR61 on mesenchymal stem cells, osteoblasts, and endothelial cells was reported (Schutze et al., 2005). Where in embryonic development, CYR61 is expressed in the placenta and cardiovascular and skeletal system (Kireeva et al., 1997; O'Brien et al., 1992). A vital role for CYR61 during embryogenesis has been reported in knockout mice that suffers embryonic death because of vascular defects in the placenta (Mo et al., 2002). Due to their early embryonic lethality, the CYR61 mutants did not show defects in skeletal development (Mo et al., 2002). Consistent with the angiogenic property of CYR61, its expression is elevated in healing wounds (Chen et al., 2009; Latinkic et al., 2001). Furthermore, CYR61 promotes chondrogenic differentiation in mouse limb bud mesenchymal micromass cultures (Wong et al., 1997). Taken together, CYR61 can act both as an angiogenic and chondrogenic factor; two characteristics that appear to be 'conflicting' since cartilage is a predominantly avascular tissue. Angiogenesis is a pivotal event in endochondral bone formation. It has been shown that hCYR61 is regulated by 1a, 25-dihydroxyvitamin D3 (1,25- (OH)2D3) and growth factors in fetal human osteoblasts (Schutze et al., 1998). Furthermore, it could be suggested that hCYR61 localizes to the secretory pathway in primary osteoblasts and fetal human osteoblasts, and it is secreted from these cells (Lechner et al., 2000).

The fact that hCYR61 exerts extracellular signaling function on endothelial cells, (Babic et al., 1998; Kolesnikova et al., 1998) simultaneously demonstrates the role of hCYR61 as an extracellular signaling molecule in human bone (Lechner et al., 2000). In a rat fracture model, (Hadjiargyrou et al., 2000) the expression of CYR61 mRNA and protein was induced during healing and the highest peak of CYR61 mRNA expression associated with chondrogenesis indicates that it may act as an important regulator of fracture healing. The CYR61 protein was detected in fibroblasts, osteoblasts, proliferating chondrocytes, and immature osteocytes, as well as in the osteoid matrix (Hadjiargyrou et al., 2000). Furthermore, a significantly reduced expression of CYR61 has been described in fibroblasts and smooth muscle cells by mechanical stress (Schell et al., 2005; Tamura et al., 2001).

The CYR61 protein expression was up-regulated at the early phase of fracture healing (2 weeks postoperative) and decreased the healing time. There were differences in the early expression of CYR61 protein between the two groups. The callus formed in the group stabilized with the semi-rigid fixator (II) which allows higher amounts of inter-fragmentary movement and thus showed a trend to a lower CYR61 protein expression at the early phase of fracture healing in comparison to the group treated with the rigid fixator (I).

Hadjiargyrou and co-workers primarily identified CYR61 to be up-regulated during fracture healing compared to intact bone (Hadjiargyrou et al., 2000). They showed that the CYR61 mRNA expression was regulated temporally in callus and that the highest expression is correlated with chondrogenesis. The mRNA expression of CYR61 during fracture repair is controlled temporally with elevated levels seen as early as PF day 3 and day 5. They increase effectively at PF day 7 and day 10, and lastly declining at PF day 14 and day 21. The CYR61 mRNA levels are approximately 10-fold greater than those detected in intact femurs. The released form of CYR61 also was observed in the newly formed osteoid with no detection in hypertrophic chondrocytes or in mature cortical osteocytes. These results imply that CYR61 plays a vital role in cartilage and bone formation and may act as an important regulator of fracture healing (Hadjiargyrou et al, 2000).

Jasmin et al., also found an up-regulation of the CYR61 protein expression during the early phase of healing in which chondrogenesis took place. This finding supports the role of CYR61 as a chondrogenic regulator. During secondary fracture healing, the cartilage formed by differentiation of mesenchymal cells into chondroblasts must be replaced by bone (endochondral ossification). Therefore, it is important that the cell differentiation occurs in a fast and regular way. Wong et al., (1997) demonstrated that the CYR61 protein promotes chondrogenesis in micromass cultures of limb bud mesenchymal cells in vitro. They showed that the CYR61 protein promotes cell aggregation, accelerates the rate of differentiation of mesenchymal cells into chondroblasts, and increases the extent of differentiation in mesenchymal cells. Jasmin et al., found a delayed and reduced expression of CYR61 protein in cartilage, probably leading to a less effective or suboptimal chondrocyte differentiation and therefore to a longer persistence of cartilage in callus. Thus, they demonstrate that the CYR61 protein may play an important role during chondrogenesis in fracture healing.

4

Material and Method

Present section deals with the detailed approaches, techniques and analytical parameters used for collection, analysis and explanation of the various parameters in the enrolled patients. In this section we have described the selection of patients and also the protocols of various experiments used for the fulfillment of various objectives proposed in the study.

4.1   Study Area

The study was conducted in Department of Orthopaedic Surgery/Department of Biochemistry, King George's Medical University, Lucknow, U.P.

4.2   Study Design

The present study was a prospective cohort study.

4.3   Sample Size

Assuming 97% prevalence of union in tibial bone (Malekpoor et al. 2009) and by taking 80% power and 5% significance level, the calculated sample size was 47. Considering 15% loss to follow-up, the final sample size was 55. Sample size was calculated using the formula:

$$Sample\ Size = \frac{4pq}{d^2},$$

where, p = prevalence of union; d = assumed difference (0.05); q = (1–p).

4.4   Inclusion Criteria

Simple fresh (< 3rd days) traumatic diaphyseal fractures of tibia managed conservatively in either males or females of more than 18 years and less than 40 years.

4.5   Exclusion Criteria

i.   Age < 18 years or > 40 years. (After 40 years, Osteoporotic changes may occur).

ii.   Polytrauma.

iii. Patients with known osteoporosis.

iv. Patients with known metabolic diseases such as hypothyroidism.

v.   Pathological fracture.

vi. Compound fracture.

vii. Patients with known liver or renal dysfunctions

viii. Immuno-compromised patients.

ix. Single tibial fracture with intact fibula.

x.   Patients managed surgically.

xi. Patients coming after third post-fracture days.

xii. Malnourished.

xiii. Patient not willing.

4.6   Study Protocol

All patients included in this study were managed conservatively (reduction -setting and above knee plaster cast under general/regional anesthesia).

Prior to the management, the clinical and radiological examinations were done by principal investigator/Co-investigator. The clinical examination included observations such as skin condition, abnormal mobility, bony tenderness. The radiological examination was done by plain x-rays (antero- posterior and lateral view) done by x-ray machine (Allangers 525 (500mA)) at 25mAs, 65KVP and at 2.5 feet FFD at trauma center. No digital x-ray was done in any case. The basic sign of fracture bones of leg was pain, swelling, inability to walk or bear weight on the leg with break in continuity of both bones of leg with or without displacement radiologically. To exclude malnourished patients, the nutritional examination like Hemoglobin percentage (manually), Serum albumin (ELITech Clinical System), and Serum ferritin (Roche Analyser) were done at Department of Biochemistry. The baseline (at 04th post-fracture day) biochemical marker examination was carried out in enrolled patients for Cysteine Rich Angiogenic Inducer 61 (CYR61) from their 3ml venous blood. The Glyceraldehyde 3-phosphate dehydrogenase (GAPDH) used as an internal control. The peripheral blood (3ml) was collected into EDTA (1ml) and plain vials (2ml), than the biochemical examination was done quantitatively both at mRNA and protein level at 4th post-fracture day. They were admitted for next 24–48 hours and then discharged with a standard advice written on discharge card by principal investigator/Co-investigator. They were regularly followed up as per following protocol:

4.6.1   Clinical Examination Follow up

At 06 weeks AKPOP (above knee plaster) was removed and splintages were given. As per clinical and radiological progress as adjudged by guide & co-guides decided that that whether above knee plaster cast (AKPOP) with walking iron or PTBPOP (patella weight bearing plaster) with walking iron was to be given. These patients were again examined at 10th weeks, on the same clinical parameters and progress in the clinical callus/union was assessed. Further follow up & management was decided by the treating surgeons as per progression of healing.

4.6.2   Radiological Examination Follow up

The radiological examination was done at 6th, 10th, 16th, 20th, 24th week and further if required. The radiological pattern of healing was evaluated using RUST Score (Whelan et al., 2010; Sabir et al., 2014). Bony healing was evaluated separately for each cortical surface (anterior, posterior, medial and lateral). The absence of callus and a visible fracture line received 1 point; callus with a visible fracture line 2 points; and callus with no visible fracture line 3 point. From the sum of these points a final RUST score was obtained, ranging from 4 for a completely ununited fracture to 12 for a definitively united fracture. A score ≥ 7 equates to a minimum of three bridge with cortical callus, at which point a fracture is considered to be radio logically united (Whelan et al., 2010; Sabir et al., 2014) (Figure 4.1). The x-rays for RUST score were examined separately by two orthopaedic surgeons blindly and findings were noted separately (Table 4.1). The average of scores of both orthopaedic surgeons was taken for final decision/analysis.

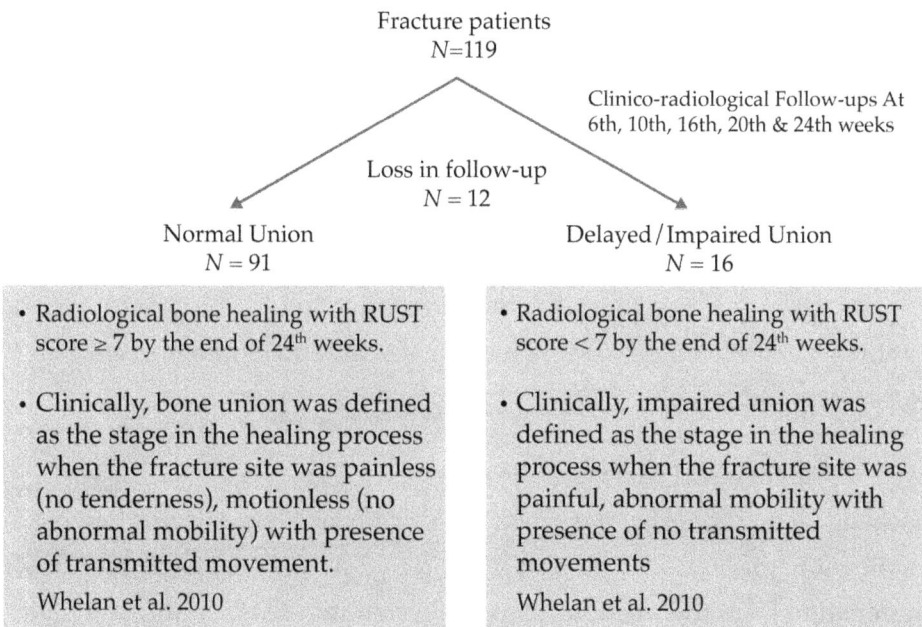

Fracture patients
N=119

Clinico-radiological Follow-ups At
6th, 10th, 16th, 20th & 24th weeks

Loss in follow-up
N = 12

Normal Union
N = 91

Delayed/Impaired Union
N = 16

• Radiological bone healing with RUST score ≥ 7 by the end of 24th weeks.

• Clinically, bone union was defined as the stage in the healing process when the fracture site was painless (no tenderness), motionless (no abnormal mobility) with presence of transmitted movement.

Whelan et al. 2010

• Radiological bone healing with RUST score < 7 by the end of 24th weeks.

• Clinically, impaired union was defined as the stage in the healing process when the fracture site was painful, abnormal mobility with presence of no transmitted movements

Whelan et al. 2010

Figure 4.1: Labeling of cases as either with Normal Healing and Impaired Healing Group at 24th week's clinic-radiological evaluation.

S no.	Weeks	Orthopedic surgeons-I	Orthopedic surgeons-II	Average RUST Score	Decision
1	6th	5	5	5	Un-united
2	10th	6	7	6.5	Un-united
3	16th	7	7	7	United
4	20th	8	9	8.5	United
5	24th	11	12	11.5	United
			Final Decision	Normal Bony Healing	

Table 4.1: Clinico-Radiological evaluation form of a patients showing normal bony healing.

These clinic-radiological evaluation at 24th week of post-fracture were used to label these healing as normal or impaired healing (may be lead to delayed/non-union). Patients with normal bony healing were defined with RUST score ≥7 by the end of 24th week along with painless (no tenderness), motionless (no abnormal mobility) with presence of transmitted movements at fracture site. However patients with impaired healing was defined as a case with RUST score <7 by the end of 24th weeks along with presence of pain, abnormal mobility with absence of transmitted movements at the fracture site (Whelan et al., 2010). Figure 4.1 deals with distribution of cases with normal and impaired healing.

At 24th week, the clinical & radiological status (RUST Score) of union was then analysed against the expression of selected biomarkers (taken at 4th, 7th, 10th, 15th and 20th post-fracture days).

4.6.3   Biochemical Marker Follow up

Biochemical marker examination (CYR61) was carried out in enrolled patients at following intervals i.e. 7th, 10th, 15th, 20th days for the biochemical marker examination from their venous blood collected into EDTA (1ml) and plain vials (2ml) both at mRNA and protein level. After the discharge, blood collection was done by the investigator at home of the patients.

4.6.3.1   Whole Blood Preparation & Storage

0.2 ml of whole blood to 0.75 ml of TRI Reagent BD (Sigma) supplemented with 20 ml of 5 N acetic acid per 0.2 ml of whole blood was added. The tube were closed and vortex to ensure that mixing is thorough. All the blood samples were in duplicates and were stored for RNA isolation at −80°C in deep freezer.

4.6.3.2   Total RNA Isolation

1. Phase Separation

To ensure complete dissociation of nucleoprotein complexes, samples were allowed to stand for 5 minutes at room temperature. Further, 0.2 ml of chloroform per 0.75 ml of TRI Reagent BD (Sigma T-3809) was added. The sample was tightly covered and shaked vigorously for 15 seconds and allowed to stand for 2-5 minutes at room temperature. The resulting mixture was centrifuged at 12,000 x g for 15 minutes at 4°C. Centrifugation separated the mixture into 3 phases: a lower red organic phase (containing protein), an interphase (containing DNA), and a colorless upper aqueous phase (containing RNA).

2. RNA Precipitation

The aqueous phase was transferred to a fresh tube through pipetting and 0.5 ml of isopropanol was added per 0.75 ml of TRI Reagent BD used for the initial lysis and mixing done. The sample allowed to stand for 5-10 minutes at room temperature and then centrifuged at 12,000 X g for 8 minutes at 4°C. The RNA precipitate formed at pellet on the side and bottom of the tube.

3. RNA Wash

The supernatant was removed and RNA pellet was washed by adding 1 ml (minimum) of 75% ethanol per 0.75 ml of TRI Reagent BD. Vortex the sample and then centrifuged at 7,500 x g for 5 minutes at 4°C.

4. RNA Solubilization

The RNA pellet was dried for 5-10 minutes by air-drying. Further, 08µl of DEPC treated water to each RNA pellet was added. To facilitate dissolution, repeated pipetting was done with a micropipette at 55–60°C for 10–15 minutes. The duplicate samples were mixed to the single one and finally the RNA concentration measured using Nanodrop.

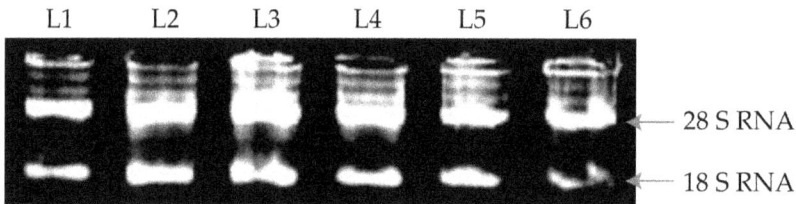

Figure 4.2: Agarose gel showing 28 S and 18 S RNA isolated from the fractured patient's blood samples in lane 1-6.

4.6.3.3   Serum Preparation

The whole blood (2ml) samples collected in the serum vials and allow the blood to clot by leaving it undisturbed at room temperature for 15-30 minutes. Then the clot was centrifuged at 1,500 x g for 10 minutes in a refrigerated centrifuge. The resulting supernatant was designated serum which was immediately transferred into a clean microcentrifuge tube. The serum was being apportioned into two aliquots and stored at –20 °C, till further going for western blotting.

4.6.3.4   Analysis of mRNA expression- Real-time PCR

1. Complementary DNA (cDNA) synthesis

The first strand of cDNA was synthesized by using GoScript™ Reverse Transcription kit (Promega) . The 20µl of reaction mixture was consisted of 2µl of 10 X RT-buffer, 2µl of dNTP mix (containing 10 mM of dNTP mix), 1µl of oligo dT primer (10 pM), 1µl of Promega RTase (4 U/µl) and heat denatured RNA. For the denaturation of RNA, 100 ng of RNA was taken in a volume of 10 µl (using RNase free water) heat denatured at 65 °C for 5 minutes and immediately snap cooled in ice. The reaction was carried out at 37 °C for 2 hours (Figure 4.3).

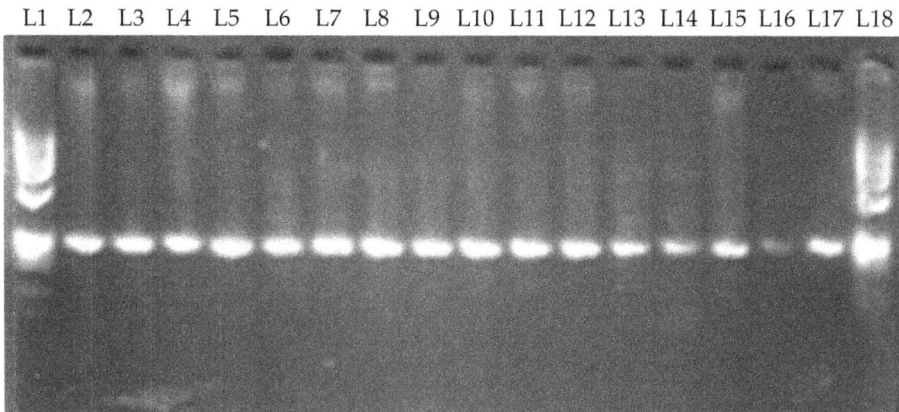

L1 L2 L3 L4 L5 L6 L7 L8 L9 L10 L11 L12 L13 L14 L15 L16 L17 L18

Figure 4.3: Agarose gel run on complementary DNA (cDNA), lane 1 & 18 with 100bp ladder and lane 2 to lane 16 with samples.

2. *Amplification of cDNA by PCR*

The cDNA was first amplified for GAPDH gene that was used as a positive control for the present study. The amplification of GAPDH gene provided the means of qualitative as well as quantitative analysis of each synthesized cDNA. To check the quality of cDNA, GAPDH was amplified by using 1 µl, 1.5 µl, 2.0 µl and 3 µl of template cDNA. The 20 µl of the PCR reaction mixture consisted of 2 µl of 10X PCR buffer, 0.25 µl of MgCl2 (25mM), 1 µl of each dNTP (10mM), 1 µl of each GAPDH primer (10 pM) and 2 units of Taq polymerase (3 U/µl). The thermal cycling condition for GAPDH gene is given in the Table 4.2.

Gene	Denaturation	Annealing	Extension
CYR61	94 °C for 5 minutes	55 °C for 45 seconds	70 °C for 5 minutes
GAPDH	95 °C for 8 minutes	58 °C for 45 seconds	70 °C for 5 minutes

Table 4.2: Details of thermal cycling conditions for RT-PCR analysis.

For the transcriptional analysis of different genes, two sets of primers were used (Table 4.3). The PCR reaction (20µl) was set by mixing 2 µl of 10 X PCR buffer, 1 µl of each dNTP (10mM), 1.0 µl of each gene primer (10 pM),

1 µl of Taq polymerase (3 U/µl) and 1 µl of cDNA. The thermal cycling condition for genes is given in Table 4.2. The normalized amount of targeted
genes was then compared using the comparative Ct-method.

Genes	Sequence	
CYR61 Cysteine-rich angiogenic inducer 61 (CYR61)		
CYR61; F Primer	TGGAGTTATATTCACAGGGTCTG	FAM-TAMRA
CYR61; R Primer	GCAGCTCAACGAGGACTG	
CYR61; Probe	CGCCGAAGTTGCATTCCAGCC	
Glyceraldehyde 3-phosphate dehydrogenase (GAPDH)		
GAPDH; F Primer	GAAGGTGAAGGTCGGAGTC	FAM-TAMRA
GAPDH; R Primer	GAAGATGGTGATGGGATTTC	
GAPDH; Probe	CAAGCTTCCCGTTCTCAGCC	

Table 4.3: List of Primers and Probes used in gene expression study.

4.6.3.5   Expression and Analysis of Proteins (Sodium dodecyl sulfate-polyacrylamide gel electrophoresis and Western blot)

1. Serum Protein Estimation

Serum protein concentrations were measured following the Bicinchoninic
acid (BCA) kit method using bovine serum albumin (BSA) as the standard.
BCA used for the colorimetric detection and quantitation of total protein.
This method involved reduction of Cu^{+2} to Cu^{+1} by protein in an alkaline me-
dium (the biuret reaction) with the highly sensitive and selective colorimetric detection of the cuprous cation (Cu^{+1}) using a reagent containing BCA.

- **BCA Reagent A:** Containing sodium carbonate, sodium bicarbonate,
  BCA and sodium tartrate in 0.1M sodium hydroxide.
- **BCA Reagent B:** Containing 4% cupric sulfate.

During serum protein estimation mix reagent A (50 part) and reagent B (1
part) and vertex properly and then add 200µl of BCA reagent to 20µl of serum protein in 96 well plate/well and kept at 37 °C for 30 min. The purple-
colored reaction product of this assay is formed by the chelation of two mol-

ecules of BCA with one cuprous ion. The intensity of color developed 30 min later, was measured at 562nm in spectrophotometer against blank samples without protein. The total protein content in the sample was calculated using BSA standard curve drawn (i.e. 6.2–8.1g/l).

	Molecular Weight (kDa)
CYR61	44
GAPDH	36

Table 4.4: Molecular weight of selected biomarker.

2. *Preparation of Samples for SDS-PAGE*

For denaturation, loading buffer with the anionic denaturing detergent SDS, and boiled the mixture at 95–100 °C for 5 minutes. The standard loading buffer is called 2X Laemmli buffer. The 2X is to be mixed in a 1:1 ratio with the sample (Appendix B).

3. *Gel electrophoresis (SDS-PAGE)*

 A sample from the initial expression was thawed and serum was dissolved in 1:1 ratio loading buffer. The samples were denatured by boiling for 7 min. Separation of the denatured serum sample were loading in 12% PAGE containing SDS and separated by electrophoresis (130 volt for 6 hrs.) and to determine the molecular weight of the sample-proteins, a protein standard molecular marker ladder 100 kDA (NEB, UK) was used for comparison. This standard was composed of a mixture of proteins with defined molecular weight. After electrophoresis the gels were stained with Coomassie blue solution. The stained gel was washed in Milli Q-water for 15 minutes before staining it with Coomassie blue protein staining solution (Fermentas, Germany). Unspecific staining was removed with Milli Q-water for a couple of hours (Figure 4.4).

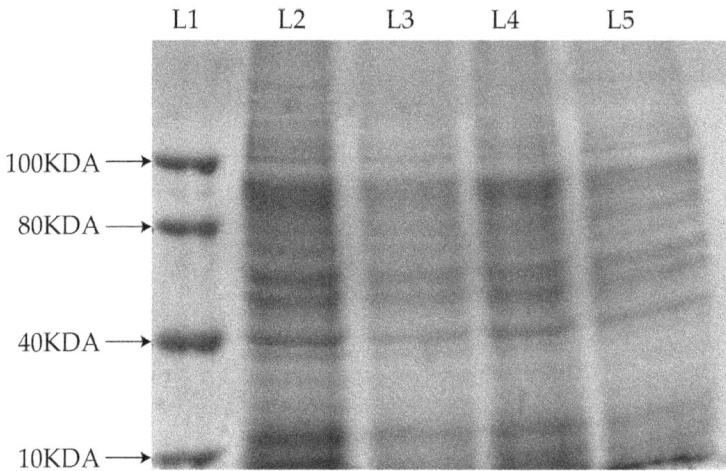

Figure 4.4: Analysis of SDS-PAGE of fractured patients. Lane 1 Molecular marker, Lane 2 to lane 5 samples.

4. *Transfer of Proteins and Staining (Western Blotting)*
*   Transfer of protein was carried out using wet transfer method. In wet transfer, the gel and membrane are sandwiched between sponge and paper (sponge/paper/gel/membrane/paper/sponge) and all are clamped tightly together after ensuring no air bubbles have formed between the gel and membrane (60 volt for 60 min).
*   Proteins were transferred on 0.2µm Nitrocellulose membrane (Sigma-Aldrich, USA).
*   To check for success of transfer, membrane was washed in mixture of Tris-Buffered Saline and Tween 20 (TBST). Membrane was further incubated on an agitator for 5 min into Ponceau Red 1:10.
*   Membrane was washed extensively in water until the water is clear and the protein bands are well- defined. The membrane was further destained completely by repeated washing in TBST.
*   Block the membrane with blocking buffer in 5% not-fat dry milk in 0.2% TBST, for 2hrs at 40 °C on shaker.
*   Rinse for 5 seconds in TBST after the incubation.
*   Incubate the membrane in primary polyclonal antibody (Cyr61(1:1000) (Santacruz Biotech, USA)) overnight at 4°C on shaker.

No.	Examinations	Work done	Time interval
1	Clinical examination	Clinical tests such as skin condition, abnormal mobility and bony tenderness were gently examined.	At admission Follow-up At 06th, 10th post-fracture weeks (Further, follow up & management was decided by the treating surgeons as per progression of healing.)
2	Radiological examination	X- ray was done and then examined separately using RUST scoring.	At admission Follow-up At 06th, 10th, 16th, 20th, 24th post-fracture weeks.
3	Biochemical marker examination (CYR61)	mRNA & Protein expression of CYR61 was quantified using Real time-PCR & Western blotting assay.	4th post-fracture days. Follow-up At 7th, 10th, 15th and 20th post-fracture days.
4	Distribution of cases into Normal Healing and Impaired Healing Groups at 24th weeks (clinical & radiological parameters)		
5	Difference in mean mRNA and protein expression of CYR61 between the Normal Healing and Impaired Healing Groups was analyzed and the peak expressions of CYR61 were correlated with RUST score at different follow-ups.		
6	Analysis and inferences.		

Table 4.5: Summary of the methodology section (* – The biochemical examination and X- ray evaluation are conducted in blinded manner as per standard protocol).

- Wash membrane 3 times with 0.2% of phosphate buffered saline supplemented with Tween 20 (PBST).
- Incubate the membrane in Horse radish peroxidase conjugated secondary antibody (1:1,000-1:-20,000; SC-2004 Goat-anti-Rabbit IgG-HRP, Santacruz Biotech, USA)

- Wash membrane 3 times with 0.2% PBST Protein bands were detected using chemiluminescent substrate (Novex HRP chromogenic substrate, Invitrogen) and were quantified using Scion Image for Windows (NIH, USA).

Time intervals	Clinical examination	Radiological examination	Biochemical marker examination
4th day	✗	✗	✓
7th day	✗	✗	✓
10th day	✗	✗	✓
15th day	✗	✗	✓
20th day	✗	✗	✓
6th week	✓	✓	✗
10th week	✓	✓	✗
16th week	✗	✓	✗
20th week	✗	✓	✗
24th week*	✗	✓	✗

Table 4.6: Follow up of different examinations (* – At 24th week: Distribution of cases into Normal and Impaired Healing Groups.)

4.7   Statistical Analysis

Statistical analysis was performed using GraphPad InStat software (version 3.05 for Windows, SanDiego, CA, USA). The demographic characteristics were compaired using between both groups was determined using Student t test (Unpaired), Fisher exact test or Chi square test. All values are expressed as mean±SD. Statistical mean significant difference in biomarker (CYR61) expression and radiological examinations in both groups was determined using Mann-Whitney U test, one-way analysis of variance (ANOVA) followed by Dunn's multiple comparisons test followed by Kruskal- Wallis Test. The correlation analysis between the clinco-radiological progression and biomarker expression were done by Spearman correlation. At 95% confidence interval, values of $p < 0.05$ were considered statistically significant.

Simple Diaphyseal Tibial Fracture
(As per inclusion/exclusion criteria)
($n = 119$)

Clinical examination	**Radiological examination**	**Biochemical marker examination (CYR61)**
Clinical tests such as skin condition, abnormal mobility and bony tenderness was be gently examined.	Plain X- ray was done to asses fracture.	Baseline (4th post-fracrure day) mRNA & protein expression of selected biomarkers was quantified using Real time-PCR & Western blotting assay.

Reduction -Setting & Above Knee Plaster
(Discharge & Follow-up)

Clinical examination:	**Radiological examination:**	**Biochemical marker examination (CYR61):**
Follow up At 6th, 10th weeks of post-fracrure (further, follow up & management was decided by the treating surgeons as per progression of union)	Follow up X-rays was done at 6th, 10th, 16th, 20th & 24th weeks of post-fracrure and then examined separately by orthopaedic surgeons/ radiologist for the progression of bony union using RUST scoring.	Follow up At 7th, 10th, 15th & 20th days of post-fracrure

Loss of follow up
($n = 12$)

Normal Union ($n = 91$) ← **At 24th week** → **Impaired Union** ($n = 16$)

The clinical & radiological status (RUST Score) of union was then analysed against the expression of selected biomarker

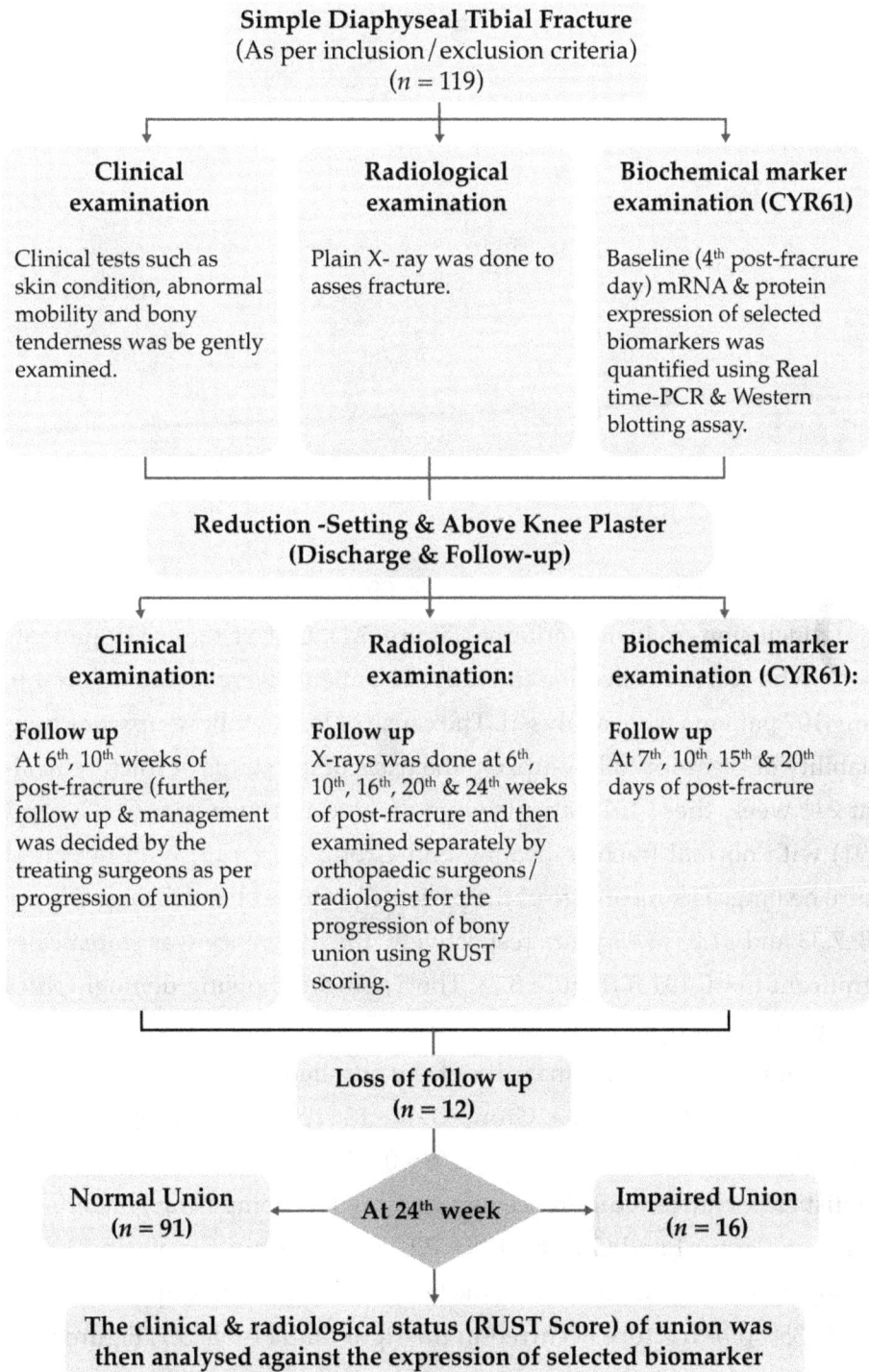

Figure 4.5: Flowchart of Methodology.

5

Observation and Results

O ut of 128 patients who are eligible, 09 patients were excluded as per inclusion-exclusion criteria (Figure 5.1). Out of these 119 patients who were enrolled in our study, 12 patients were lost to follow-up. So only 107 patients were analysed. The cause of lost to follow-ups was non-availability of cases for follow-up. On the basis of the status of fracture healing at 24th week, these 107 patients were divided into two groups: Group I ($n = 91$) with normal fracture healing and Group II ($n = 16$) with impaired fracture healing. The mean age of the patients in Group-I and Group-II were 31.08±7.33 and 31.25±6.93 years respectively, the difference was statistically insignificant ($p = 0.1313$) (Figure 5.2). The Table 5.1 showing demographics of Group-I and Group-II patients.

In both of the groups, majority of the enrolled fracture patients were male (Group-I, $n = 85$ (79.44%); Group-II, $n = 13$ (12.15%)) as compare to female (Group-I, $n = 06$ (5.61%); Group-II, $n = 03$ (2.80%)) (Table 5.1; Figure 5.3). No statistical significant difference was found while comparing gender's ratio between Group-I and Group- II ($p = 0.1313$). In Group-I, majority ($n = 50$ (46.73%)) of the fracture occurred in the left limb, whereas Group-II, majority ($n = 10$ (9.35%)) of fracture occurred in the right limb (Table 5.1; Figure 5.4). No statistical significant difference was found while comparing the side (left/right) of fracture between Group-I and Group- II ($p = 0.2785$).

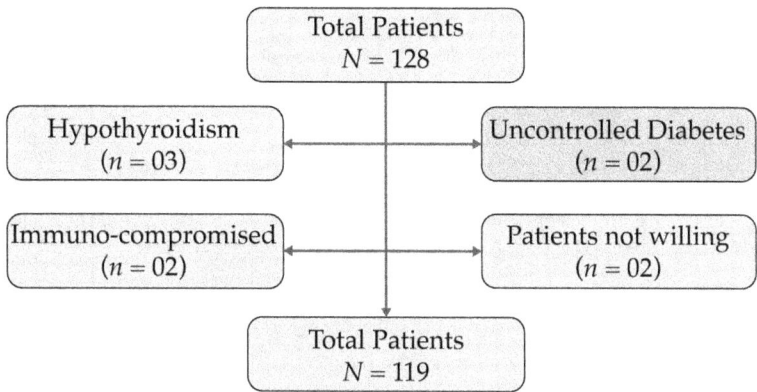

Figure 5.1: Patients enrolment as per inclusion-exclusion criteria.

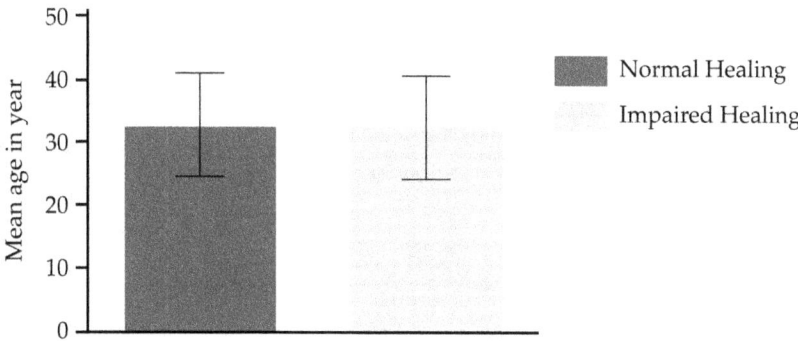

Figure 5.2: Mean age of the patients in both groups

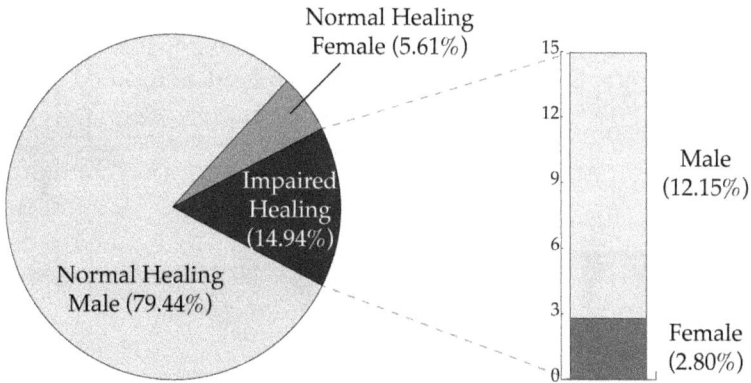

Figure 5.3: Gender distribution of patients in both groups.

Characteristic		Group I Normal Healing (*n* = 91) (85.05%)	Group II Impaired Healing (*n* = 16) (14.95%)	Significance of difference
Mean age in years±SD (range)		31.08±7.33 (18–40)	31.25±6.93 (19–40)	$t = 0.4647$; $P = 0.6431$[†]
Gender	Male	85 (79.44%)	13 (12.15%)	$P = 0.1313$[‡]
	Female	6 (5.61%)	3 (2.80%)	
Side of fracture	Left	50 (46.73%)	6 (5.61%)	$P = 0.2785$[‡]
	Right	41 (38.31%)	10 (9.35%)	
Mode of injury	Fall from height	24 (22.42%)	05 (4.67%)	$\chi^2 = 6.047$; $P = 0.1093$[‡]
	Road Traffic Accident	46 (42.99%)	07 (6.54%)	
	Simple fall	21 (19.62%)	3 (2.80%)	
	Slip on ground	0 (0)	1 (0.93%)	
AO type	A1	29 (27.10%)	4 (3.73%)	$\chi^2 = 1.246$; $P = 0.5362$[‡]
	A2	27 (25.23%)	7 (6.54%)	
	A3	35(32.71%)	5 (4.67%)	
Mean Hemoglobin±SD g/dl (range)		10.58±1.23 (8.4–13.5)	10.62±0.95 (9.4–12.3)	$t = 0.1236$; $P = 0.9019$[†]
Mean albumin level±SD g/dl (range)		3.75±0.22 (3.4–4.5)	3.66±0.16 (3.4–4.0)	$t = 1.563$; $P = 0.1212$[†]
Mean ferritin level±SD ng/ml (range)		105.19±36.6 (25–190.2)	91.81±34.2 (25–136)	$t = 1.361$; $P = 0.1765$[†]

Table 5.1: Comparison of baseline characteristics († – Student *t* test (Unpaired); ‡ – Fisher exact test; ‡ – Chi square test).

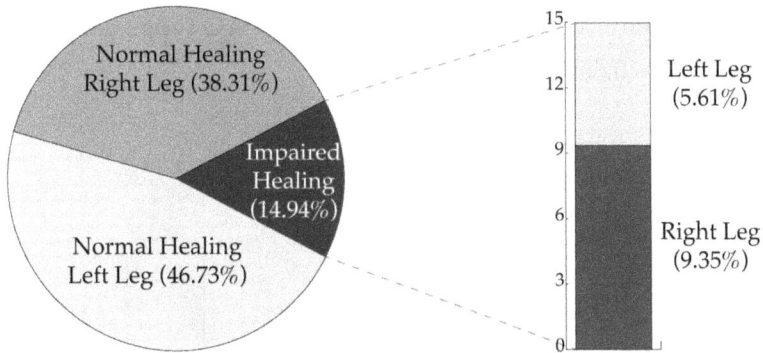

Figure 5.4: Distribution of patients according to the side of fracture in both groups.

In the present study, majority of the fracture occurred due to Road Traffic Accident (RTA) in both groups (Group-I, $n = 66$ (61.68%); Group-II, $n = 07$ (6.54%)), followed by fall from height, simple fall and due to slip on ground respectively (Table 5.1; Figure 5.5). However, statistical insignificant difference was found while comparing the mode of injury between Group-I and Group- II ($p = 0.8360$).

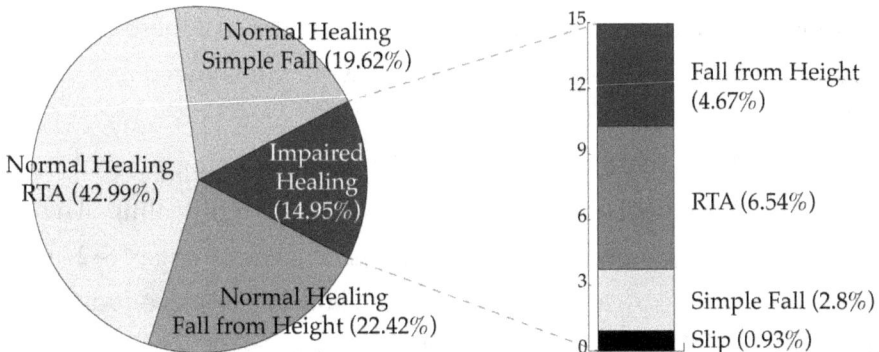

Figure 5.5: Distribution of patients according to the mode of injuries in both groups.

When these fractures were classified according to Muller's AO classi-fication, A3 in Group-I ($n = 35$ (32.71%)) and A2 in Group-II ($n = 07$ (6.54%)) are the most common one (Table 5.1; Figure 5.6). No statistical significant difference was found while comparing different AO types between Group-I and Group- II ($p = 0.6694$).

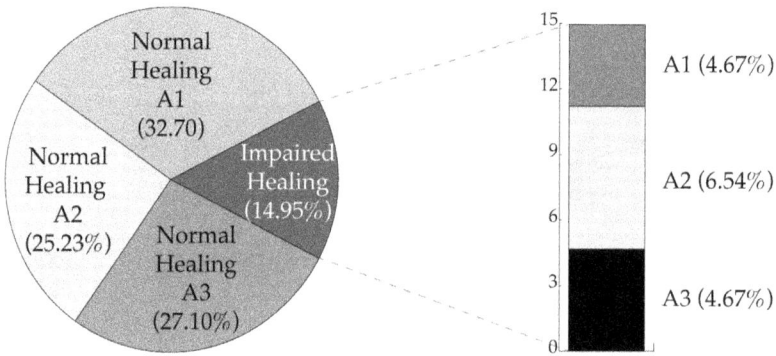

Figure 5.6: Distribution of fracture according to Mueller's Classification in both groups.

In nutritional examination of the enrolled cases, mean hemoglobin, serum albumin and serum ferritin level were 10.58±1.23 g/dl, 3.75±0.22 g/dl and 105.19±36.6 ng/ml respectively in Group-I and 10.62±0.95 g/dl, 3.66±0.16 g/dl and 91.81±34.2 ng/ml respectively in Group-II (Table 5.1; Figure 5.7, 5.8, 5.9). None of patients was excluded on this parameter. All these baseline values of the patients in Group-I and Group-II were not showed any statistical significant difference ($p > 0.05$) (Table 5.1).

In our study there were 91 (85.05%) cases showing normal fracture healing however 16 (14.95%) cases were with impaired healing. The mean time of healing in Group-I patients was 17.2±3.7 weeks (range 16–24 week).

Mean RUST score at 06th, 10th, 16th, 20th, and 24th weeks of post fracture follow-up were 6.32±0.49, 7.89±0.46, 8.41±0.60, 10.22±0.90 and 11.08±0.86 respectively in Group-I (Normal Healing) and 4.34±0.39, 4.65±0.43, 5.06±0.47, 5.62±0.46, 5.87±0.59 respectively in Group-II (Impaired Healing). Statistically significant difference (P < 0.0001) in mean RUST score were found at each radiological follow-up between Group-I and Group-II (Table 5.2; Figure 5.10).

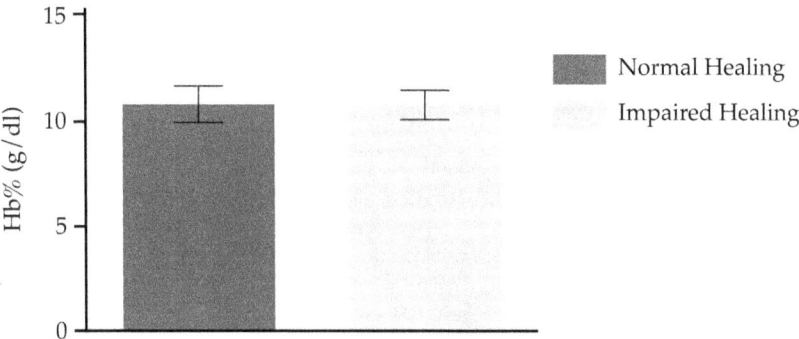

Figure 5.7: Mean hemoglobin percentage of the patients in both groups

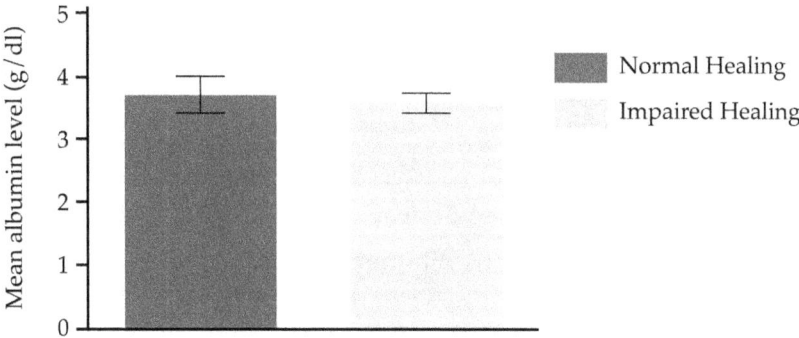

Figure 5.8: Mean serum albumin level of the patients in both groups.

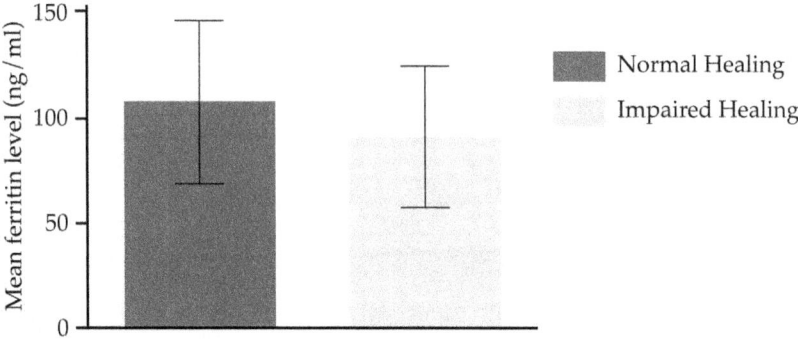

Figure 5.9: Mean serum ferritin level of the patients in both groups.

Follow-ups	RUST Score Mean±SD (Range)		95% confidence interval	P-value (two-tailed)
	Group I Normal Healing (n = 91)	Group II Impaired Healing (n = 16)		
6th week	6.32±0.49 (5.00–7.00)	4.34±0.39 (4.00–5.00)	5.17–5.48	U = 1.50; P < 0.0001*
10th week	7.89±0.46 (6.00–8.00)	4.65±0.43 (4.00–5.00)	6.10–6.43	U = 0.00; P < 0.0001*
16th week	8.41±0.60 (7.00–10.00)	5.06±0.47 (4.00–5.00)	6.54–6.92	U = 0.00; P < 0.0001*
20th week	10.22±0.90 (7.00–11.50)	5.62±0.46 (5.00–6.00)	7.72–8.13	U = 0.00; P < 0.0001*
24th week	11.08±0.86 (8.00–12.00)	5.87±0.59 (5.00–6.00)	8.23–8.72	U = 0.00; P < 0.0001*

Table 5.2: Mean RUST Score between normal and impaired healing patients (*: Significant; Mann- Whitney U test).

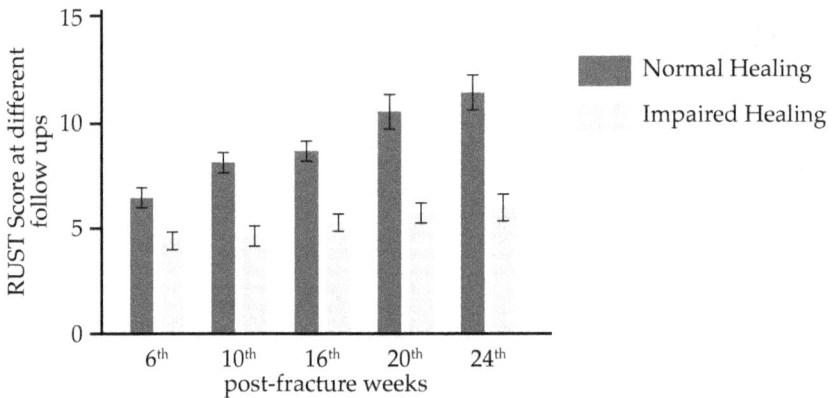

Figure 5.10: Graph showing mean RUST score between normal and impaired healing patients.

Mean RUST score at different radiological follow-ups in most of the cases within Group-I and Group-II also showed statistically significant difference (ANOVA-Dunn's Multiple Comparisons Test). Similarly, Kruskal-Wallis Test (ANOVA) also showed statistically significant difference while analysing the median of RUST score at different follow-ups within Group-I and Group-II (< 0.0001) (Table 5.3).

ANOVA (Dunn's Multiple Comparisons Test)	RUST Score Group I Normal Healing (N = 91)		RUST Score Group II Impaired Healing (N = 16)	
	Mean Rank Difference	P value (two-tailed)	Mean Rank Difference	P value (two-tailed)
6th vs. 10th week	−113.01	< 0.001*	−11.68	> 0.05
6th vs. 16th week	−163.36	< 0.001*	−26.96	> 0.05
6th vs. 20th week	−279.67	< 0.001*	−44.34	< 0.001*
6th vs. 24th week	−337.29	< 0.001*	−50.14	< 0.001*
10th vs. 16th week	−50.35	> 0.05	−15.28	> 0.05
10th vs. 20th week	−166.66	< 0.001*	−32.65	< 0.01*
10th vs. 24th week	−224.29	< 0.001*	−38.46	< 0.001*
16th vs. 20th week	−116.31	< 0.001*	−17.37	> 0.05
16th vs. 24th week	−173.93	< 0.001*	−23.18	> 0.05
20th vs. 24th week	−57.62	> 0.05	−5.81	> 0.05

Table 5.3: Mean RUST Score within normal and impaired healing patients (ANOVA) (* – Significant; † – In addition, Kruskal- Wallis Test (ANOVA) also find statistically significant difference (< 0.0001)).

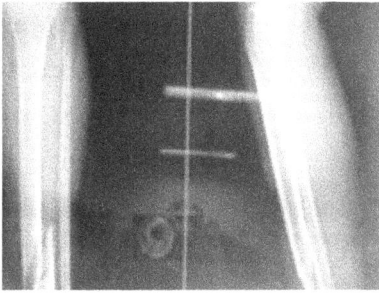
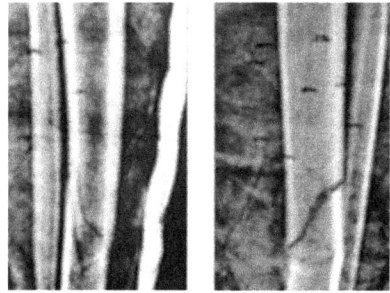

Pre-OP   Post-OP

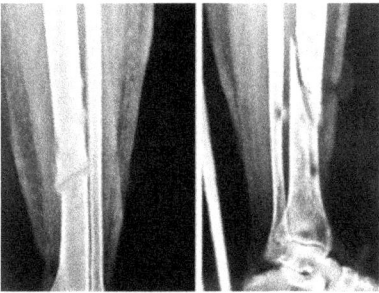
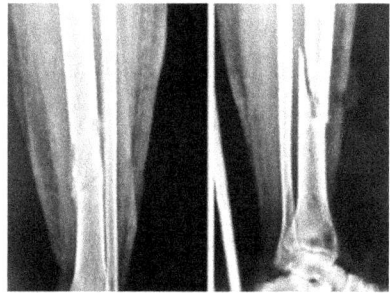

6th Week; RUST score = 05   10th Week; RUST score = 06

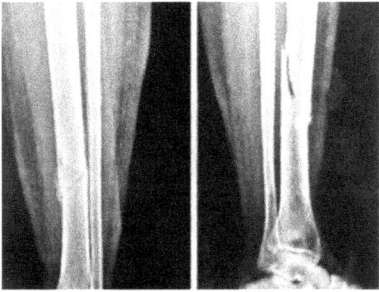
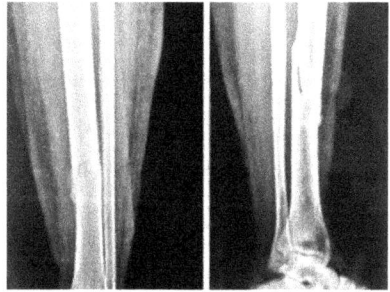

16th Week; RUST score = 07   20th Week; RUST score = 08

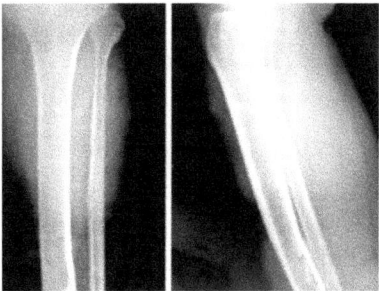

24th Week; RUST score = 11

Figure 5.11A: Radiological evaluation of healing progression using RUST scoring during follow-up for normal healing.

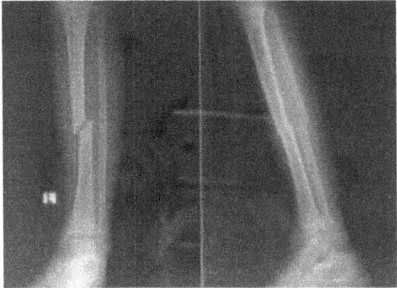
Pre-OP; RUST score = 04

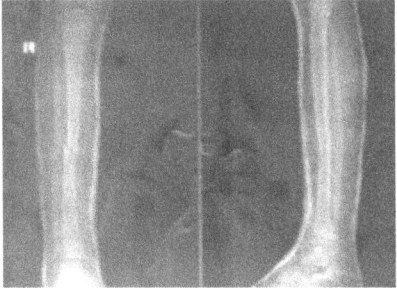
Post-OP; RUST score = 04

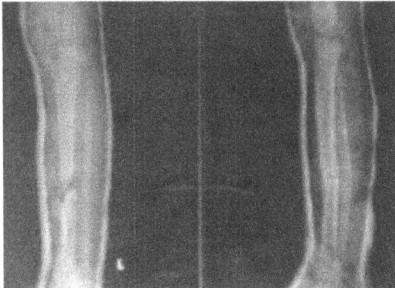
6th Week; RUST score = 04

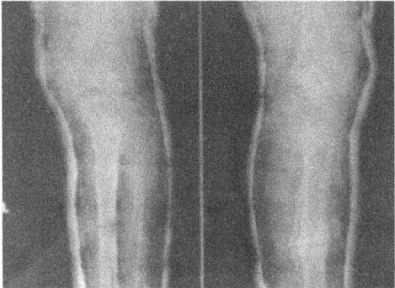
10th Week; RUST score = 05

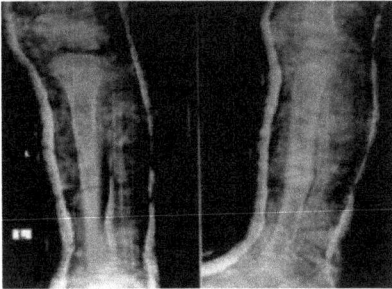
16th Week; RUST score = 05

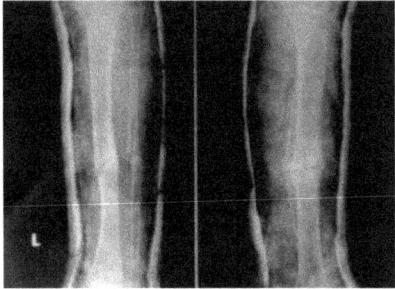
20th Week; RUST score = 05

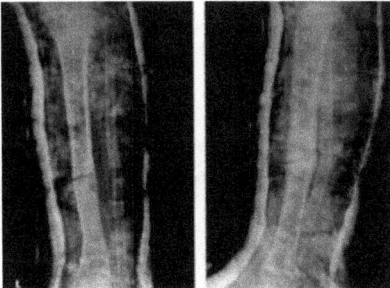
24th Week; RUST score = 06

Figure 5.11B: Radiological evaluation of healing progression using RUST scoring during follow-up for impaired healing.

In both groups, expressions of CYR61 mRNA gradually up-regulated from the beginning to the end of the post-fracture biochemical follow up. Mean CYR61 mRNA expressions at 4th, 7th, 10th, 15th and 20th days of post fracture biochemical follow-up were 2.42±0.43, 3.48±0.47, 5.21±0.50, 7.29±0.69 and 9.36±1.03 respectively in Group-I and 2.19±0.38, 3.10±0.49, 4.79±0.55, 6.69±0.93 and 8.73±1.01 respectively in Group-II. The peak of expression of CYR61 mRNA was observed at 20th day of post-fracture. The CYR61 mRNA expressions Group-I were higher at all follow-up in comparison to Group-II. While analyzing the mRNA expressions of CYR61 between Group-I and Group-II, significant statistical difference was observed at 7th, 10th, 15th and 20th post-fracture biochemical follow-up days (Table 5.4, Figure 5.12).

Follow-ups	CYR61 Mean fold change±SD (Range)		95% confidence interval	P-value (two-tailed)
	Group I Normal Healing (N = 91)	Group II Impaired Healing (N = 16)		
4th Day	2.42±0.43 (2.01–3.56)	2.19±0.38 (1.41–2.62)	2.12–2.42	U = 523.00; P = 0.0741
7th Day	3.48±0.47 (2.23–4.65)	3.10±0.49 (2.57–4.23)	1.08–2.45	U = 497.00; P = 0.0410*
10th Day	5.21±0.50 (3.87–5.98)	4.79±0.55 (3.32–5.81)	1.06–2.39	U = 501.00; P = 0.0438*
15th Day	7.29±0.69 (5.43–9.03)	6.69±0.93 (5.51–8.54)	6.67–7.31	U = 432.00; P = 0.0099*
20th Day	9.36±1.03 (6.38–10.82)	8.73±1.01 (7.45–10.93)	8.66–9.41	U = 414.50; P = 0.0063*

Table 5.4: Mean CYR61 mRNA expressions level between normal and impaired healing patients (* – Significant, Mann-Whitney U test).

Similar to CYR61 mRNA temporal expressions, the CYR61 protein expressions also gradually up-regulated from the beginning to the end of the biochemical follow up. Mean CYR61 protein expressions at 4th, 7th, 10th, 15th,

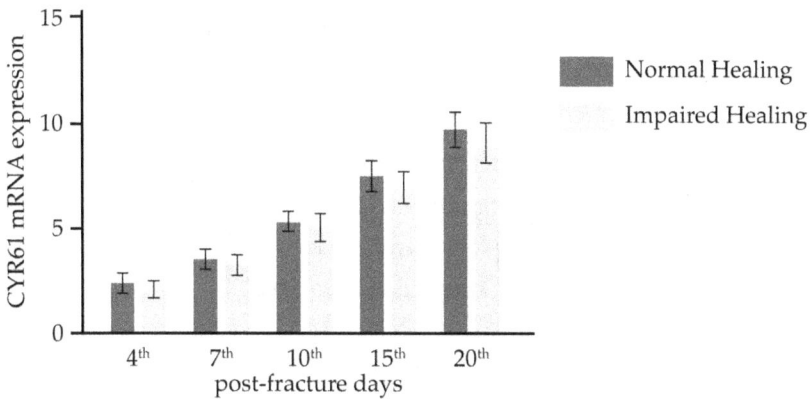

Figure 5.12: Graph showing mean CYR61 mRNA expressions level between normal and impaired healing patients.

and 20th days of post fracture biochemical follow-up were 0.40 ± 0.18, 0.67 ± 0.21, 1.31 ± 0.33, 1.68 ± 0.35 and 2.01 ± 0.43 respectively in Group-I and 0.33 ± 0.14, 0.50 ± 0.27, 1.07 ± 0.31, 1.42 ± 0.41 and 1.67 ± 0.59 respectively in Group-II. The peak of expression of CYR61 protein was obtained at 20th post-fracture day. The CYR61 protein expressions were higher at all biochemical follow up in Group-I as compared to Group-II, which showed significant statistical difference at 7th, 10th, 15th and 20th post-fracture biochemical follow-up days (Table 5.5, Figure 5.13, 5.14).

Mean CYR61 mRNA expressions at all biochemical follow ups within Group-I and at most of the follow ups in Group-II also showed statistically significant difference (ANOVA-Dunn's Multiple Comparisons Test). Similarly, Kruskal-Wallis Test (ANOVA) also showed statistically significant difference while analysing the median of CYR61 mRNA expressions at different biochemical follow-ups within Group-I and Group-II (< 0.0001) (Table 5.6).

Similar to mean CYR61 mRNA expressions, CYR61 protein expressions were also showed statistically significant differences at most of the biochemical follow up within Group-I and Group-II (ANOVA-Dunn's Multiple Comparisons Test). Similarly, Kruskal-Wallis Test (ANOVA) also showed statistically significant difference while analysing the median of

CYR61 protein expressions at different biochemical follow-up within Group-I and Group-II (< 0.0001) (Table 5.7).

Follow-ups	CYR61 Mean fold change±SD (Range)		95% confidence interval	P-value (two-tailed)
	Group I Normal Healing (N = 91)	Group II Impaired Healing (N = 16)		
04th Day	0.40±0.18 (0.03–0.76)	0.33±0.14 (0.04–0.53)	0.31–0.42	U = 582.00; P = 0.2037
07th Day	0.67±0.21 (0.28–1.37)	0.50±0.27 (0.16–1.12)	0.51–0.70	U = 492.50; P = 0.0424*
10th Day	1.31±0.33 (0.67–1.97)	1.07±0.31 (0.58–1.76)	1.09–2.77	U = 501.00; P = 0.0471*
15th Day	1.68±0.35 (1.04–2.55)	1.42±0.48 (0.93–2.44)	1.38–1.71	U = 422.00; P = 0.0076*
20th Day	2.01±0.43 (1.31–2.99)	1.67±0.59 (0.97–2.55)	1.64–2.04	U = 502.50; P = 0.0494*

Table 5.5: Mean CYR61 protein expressions level between normal and impaired healing patients (* – Significant, Mann-Whitney U test).

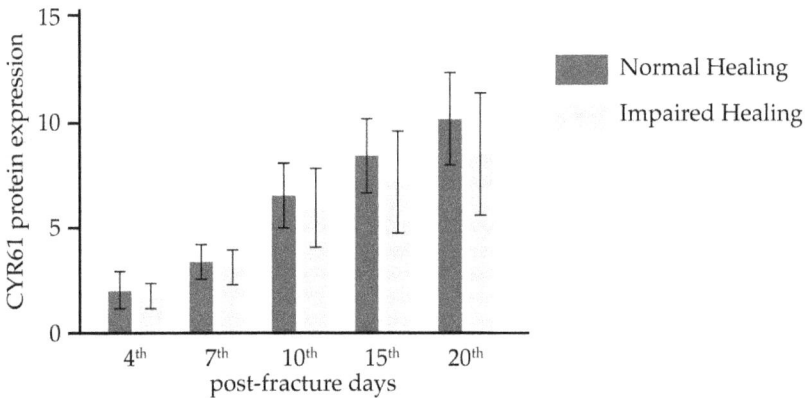

Figure 5.13: Graph showing mean CYR61 protein expressions level between normal and impaired healing patients.

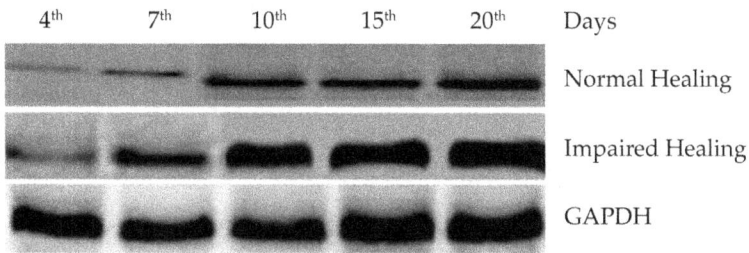

Figure 5.14: Western blot analysis of CYR61 protein expressions level between normal and impaired healing patients.

ANOVA (Dunn's Multiple Comparisons Test)	CYR61 Group I Normal Healing (N = 91)		CYR61 Group II Impaired Healing (N = 16)	
	Mean Rank Difference	P value (two-tailed)	Mean Rank Difference	P value (two-tailed)
4th day vs. 7th day	−82.46	< 0.001*	−15.93	> 0.05
4th day vs. 10th day	−176.51	< 0.001*	−31.31	< 0.01*
4th day vs. 15th day	−274.00	< 0.001*	−48.68	< 0.001*
4th day vs. 20th day	−352.50	< 0.001*	−62.50	< 0.001*
7th day vs. 10th day	−94.04	< 0.001*	−15.37	> 0.05
7th day vs. 15th day	−191.54	< 0.001*	−32.75	< 0.001*
7th day vs. 20th day	−270.04	< 0.001*	−46.56	< 0.001*
10th day vs. 15th day	−97.49	< 0.01*	−17.37	> 0.05
10th day vs. 20th day	−175.99	< 0.001*	−31.18	< 0.01*
15th day vs. 20th day	−78.50	< 0.001*	−13.81	> 0.05

Table 5.6: Mean serum CYR61 mRNA expressions level within normal and impaired healing patients (ANOVA) (* – Significant; † – In addition, Kruskal- Wallis Test (ANOVA) also find statistically significant difference (< 0.0001)).

ANOVA (Dunn's Multiple Comparisons Test)	CYR61 Group I Normal Healing (N = 91)		CYR61 Group II Impaired Healing (N = 16)	
	Mean Rank Difference	P value (two-tailed)	Mean Rank Difference	P value (two-tailed)
4th day vs. 7th day	−61.11	< 0.05*	−11.03	> 0.05
4th day vs. 10th day	−191.59	< 0.001*	−36.81	< 0.001*
4th day vs. 15th day	−262.13	< 0.001*	−43.78	< 0.001*
4th day vs. 20th day	−310.02	< 0.001*	−49.00	< 0.001*
7th day vs. 10th day	−130.48	< 0.001*	−25.78	< 0.05*
7th day vs. 15th day	−201.02	< 0.001*	−32.75	< 0.001*
7th day vs. 20th day	−248.91	< 0.001*	−37.96	< 0.001*
10th day vs. 15th day	−70.53	< 0.01*	−6.96	> 0.05
10th day vs. 20th day	−118.43	< 0.001*	−12.18	> 0.05
15th day vs. 20th day	−47.89	> 0.05	−5.21	> 0.05

Table 5.7: Mean serum CYR61 protein expressions level within normal and impaired healing patients (ANOVA) (* – Significant; † – In addition, Kruskal- Wallis Test (ANOVA) also find statistically significant difference (< 0.0001).

Significant positive correlation was found between the peak mean CYR61 mRNA expressions level (at 20th day) and the fracture healing progression measured using RUST scoring at only 16th , 20th & 24th post-fracture week (Table 5.8, Figure 5.15).

Similarly, the peak mean CYR61 protein expressions level (at 20th day) was significantly correlated with the fracture healing progression measured using RUST scoring at 16th , 20th and 24th post-fracture week (Table 5.9, Figure 5.16).

CYR61 mRNA expression at 20th Day Versus	RUST Score at week 6	RUST Score at week 10	RUST Score at week 16	RUST Score at week 20	RUST Score at week 24
Spearman r	0.1632	0.1377	0.2347	0.4056	0.3679
95% confidence interval	−0.03319 to 0.3474	−0.05927 to 0.3243	0.04123 to 0.4111	0.2283 to 0.5568	0.1859 to 0.5254
P value (two-tailed)	0.0930	0.1574	0.0150*	< 0.0001*	< 0.0001*

Table 5.8: Correlation between the peak mean CYR61 mRNA expression level (at 20th day) with the healing progression at different follow ups (RUST Score; * – Significant).

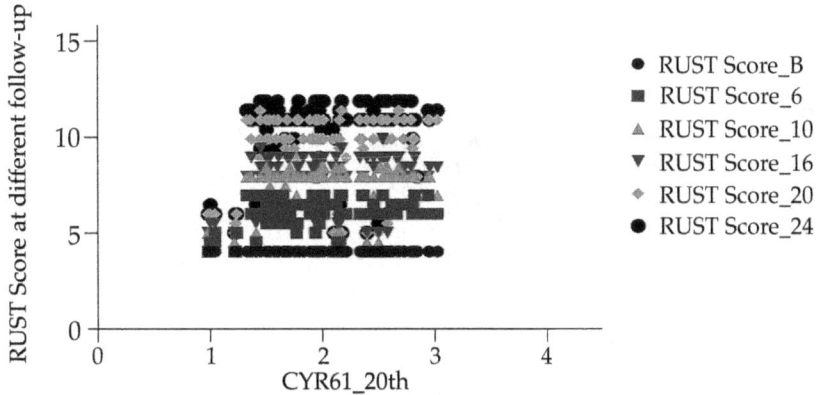

Figure 5.15: Graph showing correlation between the peak mean CYR61 mRNA expression level (at 20th day) with the healing progression at different follow ups (RUST Score).

CYR61 mRNA expression at 20th Day Versus	RUST Score at week 6	RUST Score at week 10	RUST Score at week 16	RUST Score at week 20	RUST Score at week 24
Spearman r	0.1457	0.1650	0.2350	0.2353	0.2378
95% confidence interval	−0.05111 to 0.3316	−0.03138 to 0.3490	0.04162 to 0.4115	0.04125 to 0.4113	0.04457 to 0.4139
P value (two-tailed)	0.1344	0.0895	0.0148*	0.0149*	0.0136*

Table 5.9: Correlation between the peak mean CYR61 protein expression level (at 20th day) with the healing progression at different follow ups (RUST Score; * – Significant).

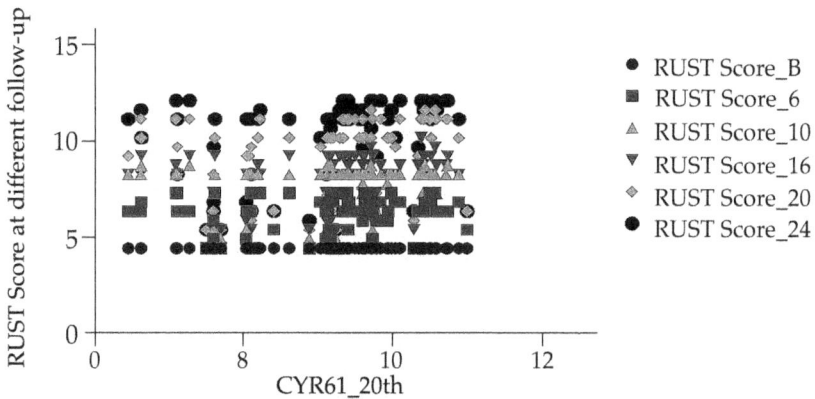

Figure 5.16: Graph showing correlation between the peak mean CYR61 protein expression level (at 20th day) with the healing progression at different follow ups (RUST Score).

6

Discussion and Conclusion

The basic aim of this study was to quantify the expression of biochemical marker (CYR61) in blood at the initial phase of fracture healing and to correlate their expression levels at regular intervals with the healing outcome of the tibial fracture. Present study focuses on the clinico-radiologically recognized impaired fracture healing in simple diaphyseal fractures of tibia and serial expression levels of CYR61. As per available literature, many studies have revealed a significant impact of CYR61 expression in the healing outcome of tibial fractures. However, no clinical studies are available which could prove the significance of biomarkers in human population. Our research hypothesis was that the fracture healing is a complex phenomenon that comprise of different overlapped but sequential biological events in which the process of angiogenesis occurs at initial stage. Therefore, it might happen that biochemical marker (CYR61) that play essential role in processes like angiogenesis may show an optimum differential expression pattern throughout the healing phase of the fracture. Any quantifiable alteration in their expression may predict early impaired fracture healing.

Amongst long bones, shaft of tibia is one of the commonest bones that is prone to fracture involving relatively higher incidence of impaired healing at the fracture site. Such impaired healing is because of lesser soft tissue coverage as it is a subcutaneous bone on anterior aspect (Patel, 2009; Reed and Mormino, 2008). The afore mentioned reason account for a high rate of tibial non unions, amounting to 2–10% of all tibial fractures which lead to significant patient morbidity (Phieffer and Goulet, 2006; Marsh, 1998; Praemer et al., 1992). Apart from the reasons mentioned earlier, other factors contributing to fracture nonunion are as follows: soft tissue damage, inadequate mechanical stability, open fractures, administration of pharmacological agents such as NSAIDs, smoking, and so on (Brinker, 2003; Giannoudis et al., 2000). Adequacy of vascular supply to the fracture site is an essential prerequisite for healing process. Inadequate vascular supply results in delayed/nonunion (Hausman et al., 2001). Despite of all optimized conditions, fracture shaft of tibia frequently develops nonunion. This tendency of fracture may reflect the role of some major biochemical events involved in the process of bone regeneration and fracture repair at molecular level. These events can be studied by analyzing expression of CYR61 for these events. As per the 24th week of clinic-radiological follow up, patients were divided into two groups; Group-I (N = 91) consisted of the normal fracture healing and Group-II (N = 16) comprised of impaired healing.

In the present study, the difference in demographic data like mean age, gender, side of fracture, Muller's AO classification and mode of injuries of the patients in Group-I (Normal Healing) and Group-II (Impaired Healing) were found to be statistically insignificant. This observation suggested that the impaired healing outcome of fracture tibial bone was independent of age, gender, mode of injuries and side as well as pattern of fracture. In the present study the nutritional examination, such as mean hemoglobin, serum albumin and serum ferritin level in Group-I and Group-II did not exhibit any statistical significant difference. However we found that commonest mode of injury was due to RTA in both groups. This finding was consistent with the observations of Bihani et al. (2016); Shah et al. (2014). In the present study majority of the cases were male (91.5%) that showed similarity with Chua et al. (2012) study in which they enrolled 91.3% male cases.

The CYR61 gene is key indicative molecule involved in angiogenesis that is prerequisite for the initiation of fracture healing. Insufficient blood supply or angiogenesis is likely to result in fracture healing impairment (Hausman et al., 2001; Haper et al., 1999).

In previous studies, it has been found that the CYR61 is an extracellular signaling molecule in human bone (Lechner et al., 2000; Babic et al., 1998; Kolesnikova et al., 1998). According to Wong et al. (1997), CYR61 acts as a novel player in chondrogenesis. O'Brien et al. (1992) also suggest that CYR61 may be important for the normal growth, differentiation or morphogenesis of the cartilaginous skeleton of the embryo.

In the present study, we observed that the expression of CYR61 mRNA as well as protein gradually up-regulated from its baseline value (i.e expression on post-fracture 4th day) till last biochemical follow-up (20th post-fracture day) in both groups. The peak expression of both CYR61 mRNA (approximately nine fold) and protein (approximately two fold) was observed at 20th post-fracture day in both groups. In comparison to Group-II, CYR61 mRNA and protein expressions were remains higher in Group-I at all biochemical follow-ups (i.e. at 04th, 07th, 10th, 15th, and 20th post-fracture day). While analyzing the CYR61 mRNA and protein expression using Mann-Whitney U test, statistical significant difference was observed between both groups at all biochemical follow-ups except at baseline value (i.e. at 4th post-fracture day). When ANOVA was applied at mean mRNA and protein expression level at different follow-ups within Group-I as well as Group-II, significant increase in CYR61 mRNA as well as protein expression was found at majority of follow-ups within each group. A positive correlation was found between peak mean value of CYR61 mRNA as well as protein expression with RUST score at 16th, 20th and 24th weeks of radiological follow-up.

To the best of our limited knowledge, no clinical study was done that could showed a correlation of simple diaphyseal tibial fracture healing outcome with to serial estimation of CYR61 gene (mRNA and protein). However, two animal studies done by Hadjiargyrou et al. and Jasmin et al. respectively had analyzed tibial fracture healing outcome in relation to serial expression of CYR61.

Hadjiargyrou et al. (2000) observed that the mRNA expression of CYR61 during fracture repair was temporally expressed in rats. Elevated level of CYR61 is seen as early as 3 and 5 post-fracture day. It rises dramatically at 7 and 10 post-fracture, and finally declines at post-fracture 14 and 21 days. These results suggest that CYR61 plays a significant role in cartilage and bone formation and may serve as an important regulator of fracture healing. In another experimental study carried out by Jasmin et al. (2005) quantified the expression of CYR61 protein during fracture healing in an Ovine tibial model. According to them CYR61 protein expressed during early phase of fracture healing is indicative to play a significant role in cartilage and bone formation. Its expression, generally up-regulated at the early phase of fracture healing (2 weeks) and then decreases over the healing time. Decreased fixation stability was associated with a reduced up-regulation of the CYR61 protein expression and a reduced vascularization at 2 weeks leading to a slower healing.

In the present study, we also found the similar gradual increase in CYR61 expression in the post-fracture follow-ups. This may prove the role of CYR61 in early angiogenesis as well as chondrogenesis in human subjects also. Though we could not observe any decline of expression by end of 20th post-fracture day. It might be probably due to the reason that the previous studies were carried out in small animal model which have shorter healing time as compare to human beings. Therefore, we may assume to observe the same decline pattern of CYR61 expression in due follow-up.

As our finding showed significant statistical difference of CYR61 mRNA as well as protein expression between both groups at 07th, 10th , 15th and 20th post-fracture days, it might be play as an prognostic biomarker to predict impaired healing early by quantifying CYR61 mRNA and protein expression level in patient peripheral blood at above said time interval.

RUST scoring is indicative of new bone formation at fracture site (callus). The present study was first to correlate the CYR61 expression with RUST scoring. In present study, a positive correlation was seen between peak CYR61 expression and mean RUST score at 16th, 20th and 24th post-fracture weeks. This observation suggests that expression of CYR61 can be correlated with new bone formation (callus at fracture site). We suggest that insignificant correlation of expression of CYR61 with RUST score at 06th and 10th week was because of the fact that radiological early callus appears late on conventional plain radiographs as well as may be due to circadian rhythm of bone remodeling, seasonal effects and high range of variation in CYR61 expression level.

Therefore in the present study, we were able to observed significant difference in CYR61 expression patterns at the initial healing phase of diaphyseal fracture between both groups. However, small sample size, limited biochemical follow-ups as well as single centric study was the limitation of the present study. Therefore author recommend further multicentric study with a large sample size to increase the reliability the obtained observations.

6.1   Conclusion

Fracture healing is a very complex process which involves expression of thousands of biomarkers. Since these biomarkers are derived from both cortical and trabecular bone, they may reflect the metabolic activity of the entire skeleton. Therefore, the detail exploration of the role as well as the correlation of the biomarkers with fracture healing or bone remodeling process are in demand. These markers not only may predict the impaired healing of fractured bone but may predict the same for various other skeleton disorders.

In the present study, we hypothesized that as the fracture healing is a complex phenomenon, comprising of different overlapped but sequential biological events in the process of angiogenesis occurs at the initial stage of fracture healing. Therefore, it might happen that biochemical marker (CYR61) that play essential role in above said processes may also show an optimum differential expression pattern in the healing phase of the fractured bone. Any quantifiable alteration in their expression may predict impaired fracture healing early.

Proving our study hypothesis, we were able to found differential temporal expression of CYR61, both at mRNA as well as protein level at the initial healing phase of fractured tibia at different intervals. The CYR61 expression showed significant higher expression (both at mRNA & protein level) in Group-I (Normal Healing) than Group-II (Impaired Healing), except the baseline and were significantly correlated with the healing progression of tibial fracture.

If the role of CYR61 in relation to the healing of the fracture is further proved, it may open new horizons for innovations in this field with an addition to our armamentarium to deal with complications associated with impaired fracture healing especially in tibial bone fractures. Since these biomarker measurements in peripheral blood are relatively less invasive, inexpensive, and can be repeated more often, it can also be used as an important prognostic tool for early identification of patients who are prone to impaired fracture healing in future.

Such an approach would benefit not only the patients' wellbeing but also to the entire health care system in terms of the cost implications associated with long lasting treatment interventions and hospitalization. We recommend further multi-centric study with large sample size to increase the validity, reliability, and generalizability of our observation and inferences.

Appendix

Lysis Buffer (500 ml)

0.32M Sucrose – 54.8 gms

1% Triton X – 5 ml

1mM MgCl$_2$ – 0.51 gms

12 mM Tris – 0.73 gms

Proteinase K Buffer (500 ml)

0.375 M NaCl 11.0 gm

0.12 M EDTA 22.4 gms

pH has to be 8.0. Hence adjust the pH with NaOH. Complete dissolution occurs only when the pH is close to 8.0.

Sodium Dodecyl Sulphate (10%; pH 7.2) (1000 ml)

SDS 100 gms

Water 900ml

Phenol Chloroform mixture (4:1) (for 1.0L)

Tris-HCl saturated phenol-800 ml

Chloroform-200 ml

Tris acetate EDTA (TAE) buffer (50X) (1000 ml)

Tris base 242 gm

Glacial acetic acid 57.1ml

EDTA (0.5 M) 100 ml

The stock solution was 50X and was diluted to 1X at the time of use.

Tris borate EDTA (TBE) buffer (10X) (1000ml)

EDTA (0.5M; pH 8.0) 40ml

Boric acid 55 gm

Tris Base 108 gm

The stock solution was prepared 10X and was diluted to 1X at the time of use.

All the reagents were prepared in Milli Q water.

Double dye (Bromophenol blue & xylene cyanol) (6X)

Bromophenol blue 0.25%

Xylene Cyanol 0.25%

Sucrose in water (w/v) 40%

Store at 4°C

Tris saturated phenol (800 ml)

Chloroform 200 ml

The water saturated phenol was washed with Tris buffer at pH 8.0 repeatedly until the pH of the wash fluid was 8.0. It was then layered with Tris at a pH of 8.0. The solution was then stored in dark bottles. Only the lower layer of the Tris saturated phenol was used.

Ethidium bromide (EtBr) (10 mg/ml)

Add 1 gm of ethidium bromide to 100 ml water. Stir on a magnetic stirrer for several hours. Wrap in an aluminum foil and store in the dark bottle at 4°C.

Working ethidium bromide (0.5µg/ml)

Bromophenol blue (6X)

Bromophenol blue 0.25%

Sucrose in water (w/v) 40%

Store at 4°C.

Ethylene diamine tetra acetic acid (EDTA) (0.5 M; pH 8.0) (1000ml)

EDTA 186.1gm

Water 800 ml (approx.)

Adjust pH 8 with NaOH (20g of NaOH pellets) make up the final volume and autoclave.

Acrylamide (30%) (100ml)

Acrylamide 29g

N, N"-methylenebisacrylamide

Water to 100 ml

Polyacrylamide gel (10%) (25 µl)

30% Acrylamide mix - 8.33 ml

TBE Buffer (10X) - 2.5 ml

Water- 13.95 ml

10% Ammonium per sulphate (APS)-200µl

TEMED- 20µl

Polyacrylamide gel (15%) (25 µl)

30% Acrylamide mix 12.5 ml

TBE Buffer (10X) 2.5 ml

Water 9.78 ml

10% Ammonium per sulfate (APS) 200µl

TEMED 20 µl

Polyacrylamide gel (20%) (25 µl)

30% Acrylamide mix 16.6 ml

TBE Buffer (10X) 2.5 ml

Water 5.61 ml

10% Ammonium per sulfate (APS) 200µl

TEMED 20 µl

Tris-glycine Running Buffer (1X)

25 mM Tris base

100190 mM glycine

0.1% SDS (pH; 8.3)

Transfer Buffer (1X)

25 mM Tris base

190 mM glycine

20% Methanol

Stacking gel (pH 6.8)

0.8 ml 30% acrylamide

3.65 ml ddH20

28 µl 10% SDS

0.5 ml 1 M Tris pH 6.8

28 µl 10% APS

5 µl TEMED

Membrane washing buffer

PBS plus 0.05% Tween-20

Membrane blocking buffer

PBS plus 5% non-fat milk powder

Dilution of Primers and Probes

The primers and probes (1OD each) were purchased from DNA agency USA. These were supplied in lyophilized state. The primers were diluted at a stock concentration of 200 pM / µl according to the following procedure.

Calculation of molecular weight (M) of the oligonucleotide

The total number of A, T, G and C in each primer sequence was counted. The molecular weight of A = 312.2, T = 303.2, G = 328.2 and C = 288.2. Accordingly, the molecular weight (M) was calculated:

$$M = nA \times 312.2 + nT \times 303.2 + nG \times 328.2 + nC \times 288.2$$

where, nA = number of Adenine; nT = number of Thiamin; nG = number of Guanine; nC = number of cytosine. For example, a primer with sequence:

CCC CAC AGC ACG TTT CTT G

Given that: nA = 3; nT = 5; nC = 8 and nG = 3, then:

$$M = 312.2 \times 3 + 303.2 \times 5 + 288.2 \times 8 + 328.2 \times 3$$
$$= 936.6 + 1516 + 2305.6 + 984.6$$
$$= 5742.8$$

Calculation of water to be added

1 OD = 30µg of single stranded DNA (oligonucleotide)
    = 30×10^{-6} gm
    = $30 \times 10^{-6} / M$ moles of oligo

To make a solution of conc. 1 mole/µl,

$$1 \text{ OD should be dissolved in} = \frac{30 \times 10^{-6}}{M} \mu l$$

To make 10^{12} p moles/µl,

$$\text{Water to be added} = \frac{30 \times 10^{-6}}{M} \mu l$$

To make 1 p mole/µl,

$$\text{Water to be added} = \frac{30 \times 10^{12} \times 10^{-6}}{M} \mu l$$

To make 200 p mole/µl,

$$\text{Water to be added} = \frac{30 \times 10^{-6}}{M \times 200} \mu l$$

For the oligonucleotide with a molecular weight of 5742.8

Water to be added = 150 × 1000 / M

$$= 150 \times 1000 / 5742.8 \ \mu l$$

$$= 26.12 \ \mu l$$

This reconstituted stock was aliquoted and kept at −80 °C. This was further diluted in HPLC grade water to give a final concentration of 10 pM/µl (working concentration).

Reference

1. AHRQ (Agency for Health Care Research and Quality): Introduction to the HCUP state inpatient databases (SID). Online Manual; URL: http://hcup-us.ahrq.gov/db/state/siddis t/Introduction_to_SID.pdf, Accessed 4 August 2011.

2. Allgower, M. and Spiegel, P. G. Internal fixation of fractures: evolution of concepts. Clin.Orthop. 1979, 138, 26–29.

3. Alt V, Donell ST, Chhabra A, Bentley A, Eicher A, Schnettler R: A health economic analysis of the use of rhBMP-2 in gustilo-anderson grade III open tibial fractures for the UK, germany, and france. Injury 2009, 40(12):1269–1275.

4. Ashman O, Phillips AM. Treatment of non-unions with bone defects: which option and why? Injury. 2013 Jan 31;44:S43-5.

5. Axelrad TW, Einhorn TA. Use of clinical assessment tools in the evaluation of fracture healing. Injury. 2011 Mar 31;42(3):301-5.

6. B.J Davis, P.J Roberts, C.I Moorcroft, M.F Brown, P.B.M Thomas, R.H Wade: Reliability of radiographs in defining union of internally fixed fractures, Injury, 2004,Volume 35, Issue 6, Pages 557-561.

7. Babic AM, Kireeva ML, Kolesnikova TV, Lau LF. CYR61, a product of a growth factor-inducible immediate early gene, promotes angiogenesis and tumor growth. Proc Natl Acad Sci USA 1998;95:6355– 6360.

8. Bhandari M, Guyatt G, Tornetta P 3rd, Emil H. Schemitsch, Marc Swiontkowsk, David Sanders, Stephen D. Walter. Randomized trial of reamed and unreamed intramedullary nailing of tibial shaft fractures. J Bone Joint Surg Am 2008, 90(12):2567–2578.

9. Bhandari M, Guyatt GH, Swiontkowski MF, Schemitsch EH: Treatment of open fractures of the shaft of the tibia. J Bone Joint Surg Br 2001, 83(1):62–68.

10. Bolander ME. Regulation of fracture repair by growth factors. Experimental Biology and Medicine. 1992 Jun 1;200(2):165-70.

11. Bornstein P, Sage EH. Matricellular proteins: extracellular modulators of cell function. Curr Opin Cell Biol.2002 14:608–616.

12. Brighton, C. T. and Hunt, R. M. Histochemical localization of calcium in the fracture callus with potassium pyroantimonate. Possible role of chondrocyte mitochondrial calcium in callus calcification. J. Bone Joint Surg. Am. 1986; 68(5), 703–715.

13. Brigstock DR, Goldschmeding R, Katsube KI, Lam SC, Lau LF, Lyons K, Naus C, Perbal B, Riser B. "Proposal for a unified CCN nomenclature". Mol. Pathol. 2003a, 56 (2): 127–128.

14. Brigstock DR. The CCN family: a new stimulus package. J Endocrinol. 2003b, 178:169–175.

15. Brinker MR, O'Connor DP. Ilizarov compression over a nail for aseptic femoral nonunions that have failed exchange nailing: a report of five cases. Journal of orthopaedic trauma. 2003 Nov 1;17(10):668-76.

16. Buckwalter, J. A., et al. Healing of the musculoskeletal tissues, in Rockwood and Green's Fractures in Adults(Rockwood, C. A., et al., ed.), Lippincott-Raven, Philadelphia,1996; pp. 261–304.

17. Calori GM, Albisetti W, Agus A, Iori S, Tagliabue L. Risk factors contributing to fracture non-unions. Injury. 2007 May 31;38:S11-8.

18. Calori GM, Mazza E, Colombo M, Ripamonti C, Tagliabue L. Treatment of long bone non-unions with polytherapy: indications and clinical results. Injury. 2011 Jun 30;42(6):587-90.

19. Chen C-C, Lau LF. "Functions and Mechanisms of Action of CCN Matricellular Proteins". Int. J. Biochem. Cell Biol. 2009, 41 (4): 771–783.

20. Cox G, Einhorn TA, Tzioupis C, Giannoudis PV.: Bone-turnover markers in fracture healing; J Bone Joint Surg Br. 2010 Mar;92(3):329-34.

21. Cruess, R. L. and Dumont, J. Fracture healing. Can. J. Surg. 1975, 18(5), 403–413.

22. D. Marsh, Concepts of fracture union, delayed union and nonunion. Clin. Orthop. 355S (1998), pp. 22–30.

23. Day SM, DeHeer DH. Reversal of the detrimental effects of chronic protein malnutrition on long bone fracture healing. J Orthop Trauma.2001; 15:47-53.

24. DeLacure, M. D. Physiology of bone healing and bone grafts. Otolaryngol.Clin. N. Am. 1994, 27(5), 859–874.

25. Einhorn TA, Hirschman A, Kaplan C, Nashed R, Devlin VJ, Warman J. Neutral protein-degrading enzymes in experimental fracture callus: A preliminary report. Journal of Orthopaedic Research. 1989 Nov 1;7(6):792-805.

26. Frost, H. M. The biology of fracture healing. An overview for clinicians.Part I. Clin.Orthop. 1989;248, 283–293.

27. Gelalis ID, Politis AN, Arnaoutoglou CM, Korompilias AV, Pakos EE, Vekris MD, Karageorgos A, Xenakis TA. Diagnostic and treatment modalities in nonunions of the femoral shaft. A review. Injury. 2012 Jul 31;43(7):980-8.

28. Gerstenfeld LC, Cullinane DM, Barnes GL, Graves DT, Einhorn TA. Fracture healing as a post-natal developmental process: Molecular,

spatial, and temporal aspects of its regulation. Journal of cellular bio-chemistry. 2003 Apr 1;88(5):873-84.

29. Giannoudis P, Tzioupis C, Almalki T, et al. Fracture healing in osteo-porotic fractures: is it really different? A basic science perspective. In-jury, 2007; 38, 90-9.

30. Giannoudis PV, Einhorn TA, Marsh D. Fracture healing: the diamond concept. Injury. 2007 Sep 30;38:S3-6.

31. Giannoudis PV, Faour O, Goff T, Kanakaris N, Dimitriou R. Masquelet technique for the treatment of bone defects: tips-tricks and future di-rections. Injury. 2011 Jun 30;42(6):591-8.

32. Giannoudis PV, Pountos I. Tissue regeneration: The past, the present and the future. Injury. 2005 Nov 30;36(4):S2-5.

33. Giannoudis PV, Snowden S, Matthews SJ, Smye SW, Smith RM. Tem-perature rise during reamed tibial nailing. Clinical orthopaedics and related research. 2002 Feb 1;395:255-61.

34. Glowacki, J. Angiogenesis in fracture repair. Clin.Orthop. 1998;355(Suppl), 82–S89.

35. Green E, Lubahn JD, Evans J. Risk factors, treatment, and outcomes as-sociated with nonunion of the midshaft humerus fracture. Journal of Surgical Orthopaedic Advances. 2005; 14(2):64–72

36. Grundnes, O. and Reikeras, O. The importance of the hematoma for fracture healing in rats. ActaOrthop.Scand. 1993a;64(3), 340–342.

37. Grundnes, O. and Reikeras, O. The role of hematoma and periosteal sealing for fracture healing in rats. ActaOrthop. Scand. 1993b; 64(1), 47–49.

38. Hadjiargyrou M, Ahrens W, Rubin CT.. Temporal expression of the chondrogenic and angiogenic growth factor CYR61 during fracture re-pair. J Bone Miner Res 2000; 15:1014–1023.

39. Hak DJ. Management of aseptic tibial nonunion. Journal of the Ameri-can Academy of Orthopaedic Surgeons. 2011 Sep 1;19(9):563-73.

40. Hammer R, Hammerby S and Lindholm B.Accuracy of radiological assessment of tibial shaft fractures in humans. Clin. Orth. R.R. 199 (1985), pp. 233–238.

41. Harper J, Klagsbrun M. Cartilage to bone—angiogenesis leads the way. Nat Med 1999; 5:617–618.

42. Hausman MR, Schaffler MB, Majeska RJ. Prevention of fracture healing in rats by an inhibitor of angiogenesis. Bone 2001; 29:560–564.

43. Hernigou PH, Poignard A, Beaujean F, Rouard H. Percutaneous autologous bone-marrow grafting for nonunions. J Bone Joint Surg Am. 2005 Jul 1;87(7):1430-7.

44. Holbourn KP, Acharya KR, Perbal B. "The CCN family of proteins: structure-function relationships". Trends Biochem. Sci 2008;33 (10): 461–473.

45. Hollinger, J. and Wong, M. E. The integrated processes of hard tissue regeneration with special emphasis on fracture healing. Oral Surg. Oral Med. Oral Pathol.Oral Radiol.Endodont. 1996;82(6), 594–606.

46. Jasmin Lienau, Hanna Schell, Devakara R. Epari, Norbert Schutze, Franz Jakob, Georg N. Duda, Hermann J. Bail. CYR61 (CCN1) Protein Expression during Fracture Healing in an Ovine Tibial Model and Its Relation to the Mechanical Fixation Stability.5 Dec 2005 in Wiley Inter Science .DOI 10.1002/jor.20035.

47. Jay P, Berge-Lefranc JL, Marsollier C, Mejean C, Taviaux S, Berta P. "The human growth factor-inducible immediate early gene, CYR61, maps to chromosome 1p". Oncogene 1997;14 (14): 1753–1757.

48. Johnson B, Christie J: Open tibia shaft fractures: a review of the literature. The Internet Journal of Orthopedic Surgery 2008, 9(1);5580

49. Jun JI, Lau LF "Taking aim at the extracellular matrix: CCN proteins as emerging therapeutic targets". Nature Reviews Drug Discovery 2011;10 (12): 945–63.

50. Kasturi G, Adler RA: Mechanical means to improve bone strength: ultrasound and vibration. Curr Rheumatol Rep 2011, 13(3):251–256.

51. Kireeva ML, Latinkic BV, Kolesnikova TV, et al. 1997. Cyr61 and Fisp12 are both ECM-associated signaling molecules: activities, metabolism, and localization during development. Exp Cell Res 233: 63–77.

52. Kireeva ML, Mo FE, Yang GP, et al. 1996. Cyr61, a product of a growth factor-inducible immediate early gene, promotes cell proliferation, migration, and adhesion. Mol Cell Biol 16:1326–1334.

53. Kolesnikova TV, Lau LF. Human CYR61- mediated enhancement of bFGF-induced DNA synthesis in human umbilical vein endothelial cells. Oncogene 1998;16:747–754.

54. Latinkic BV, Mo FE, Greenspan JA, et al. 2001.Promoter function of the angiogenic inducer Cyr61gene in transgenic mice: tissue specificity, inducibility during wound healing, and role of the serum response element. Endocrinology 142:2549– 2557.

55. Lau LF, Nathans D. "Identification of a set of genes expressed during the G0/G1 transition of cultured mouse cells". EMBO J 1985; 4 (12): 3145–3151.

56. Lau LF. "CCN1/CYR61: the very model of a modern matricellular protein". Cell. Mol. Life Sci. 2011; 68 (19): 3149–63.

57. Leask A, Abraham DJ. All in the CCN family: essential matricellular signaling modulators emerge from the bunker. J. Cell Sci. 2006;119 (Pt 23): 4803–4810.

58. Lechner A, Schutze N, Siggelkow H, Seufert J, Jakob F. The immediate early gene product hCYR61 localizes to the secretory pathway in human osteoblasts. Bone. 2000 ;27(1):53-60.

59. Madison, M. and Martin, R. B. Fracture healing, in Operative Orthopaedics (Chapman, M. W., ed.), Lippincott, Philadelphia, pp. 1993;221–228.

60. Marsell R, Einhorn TA. Emerging bone healing therapies. Journal of Orthopaedic Trauma. 2010; 24(Suppl 1):S4–8.

61. Marsh, D. R. and Li, G. (1999) The biology of fracture healing: optimising outcome. Br. Med. Bull. 55(4), 856–869.

62. Martinez De Albornoz P, Khanna A, Longo UG, Forriol F, Maffulli N: The evidence of low-intensity pulsed ultrasound for in vitro, animal and human fracture healing. Br Med Bull 2011, 100:39–57.

63. Matsumoto T, Mifune Y, Kawamoto A, et al. 2008. Fracture induced mobilization and incorporation of bone marrowderived endothelial progenitor cells for bone healing. J Cell Physiol 215:234–242.

64. McCloskey E V, Spector T D, Eyres K.S, Fern E D, O'Rourke N, Vasikaran S and Kanis J A.The assessment of vertebral deformity: A method for use in population studies and clinical trials: Osteoporosis International: Volume 3, Number 3, 138-147, (1993) DOI: 10.1007/BF01623275.

65. McKibbin, B. (1978) The biology of fracture healing in long bones. J. Bone Joint Surg. Br. 60B(2), 150–162.

66. Miller NC, Askew AE: Tibia fractures. an overview of evaluation and treatment. Orthop Nurs 2007, 26(4):216–223. quiz 224–5.

67. Minoo P, McCarthy JJ, Herzenberg J: Tibial nonunions. http://emedicine. medscape.com/article/1252306-overview. Updated 2009. Accessed 4 April 2011.

68. Mo FE, Muntean AG, Chen CC, et al. 2002. CYR61 (CCN1) is essential for placental development and vascular integrity. Mol Cell Biol 22:8709–8720.

69. Mohit Bihani, Krishna Sravanth P, Shardaindu Sharma, Rajneesh Sood, Fahad BH Intramedullary fixation of distal tibial fractures around diametaphysis using locked intramedullary cannulated distal tibial nail a prospective study. International Journal of Orthopaedics Sciences 2016; 2(2): 38-42

70. Muller, M. E., Allgower, M., and Willenegger, H. Technique of internal fixation of fractures. Springer-Verlag, New York. 1965

71. Nelson B. Watts. Clinical Utility of Biochemical Markers of Bone Remodeling. Clinical Chemistry. 1999; 45:8(B), 1359–1368.

72. Nolte PA, van der Krans A, Patka P, Janssen IM, Ryaby JP, Albers GH: Low-intensity pulsed ultrasound in the treatment of nonunions. J Trauma 2001, 51(4):693–702.

73. O'Brien TP, Yang GP, Sanders L, et al. 1990. Expression of cyr61, a growth factor-inducible immediate-early gene. Mol Cell Biol 10:3569–3577.

74. Pape HC, Giannoudis PV, Grimme K, et al. Effects of intramedullary femoral fracture fixation: what is the impact of experimental studies in regards to the clinical knowledge? Shock. 2002; 18(4):291–300. [PubMed: 12392270]

75. Perbal B. CCN proteins: multifunctional signalling regulators. Lancet 2004; 363:62–64.

76. Perren SM. Evolution of the internal fixation of long bone fractures. The scientific basis of biological internal fixation: choosing a new balance between stability and biology. J Bone Joint Surg Br. 2002; 84(8):1093–110.

77. Perren, S. M. Physical and biological aspects of fracture healing with special reference to internal fixation.Clin.Orthop. 1979; 138, 175–196.

78. Perren, S. M. The biomechanics and biology of internal fixation using plates and nails. Orthopedics 1989; 12(1),21–34.

79. Perren, S. M., Cordey, J., and Gautier, E. Rigid internal fixation using plates: terminology, principle and early problems, in Fracture Healing (Lang, J. M., ed.), Churchill Livingstone, New York, pp. 1987; 139–151.

80. Phieffer LS, Goulet JA. Delayed unions of the tibia. J Bone Joint Surg Am. 2006 Jan 1;88(1):205-16.

81. Praemer A, Furner S, Rice DP: Musculoskeletal conditions in the United States. Park Ridge, IL: American Academy of Orthopedic Surgeons; 1992.

82. Rahn, B. A., et al. (1971) Primary bone healing. An experimental study in the rabbit. J. Bone Joint Surg. Am. 53(4),783–786.

83. Reed LK, Mormino MA. Distal tibia nonunions. Foot and ankle clinics. 2008 Dec 31;13(4):725-35.

84. Roger Wade and James Richardson: Outcomes in fracture healing- a review, Injury, Volume 32, Issue 2, March 2001, Pages 109-114.

85. Sabir Ali, Ajai Singh, Avinash Agarwal, Anit Parihar, Abbas Ali Mahdi, Rajeshwar Nath Srivastava. Reliability Of The RUST Score For The Assessment Of Union In Simple Diaphyseal Tibial Fractures. Vol 5, No 5 (2014), DOI: http://dx.doi.org/10.7439/ijbr.v5i5.610

86. Sarmiento A, Latta L. Closed functional treatment of fractures. Springer Science & Business Media; 2012 Dec 6.

87. Schell H, Epari DR, Kassi JP, et al. 2005. The course of bone healing is influenced by the initial shear fixation stability. J Orthop Res 23:1022–1028.

88. Schenk R, Willenegger H. Morphological findings in primary fracture healing. InSymp Biol Hung 1967 (Vol. 7, pp. 75-86).

89. Schenk R, Willenegger H. On the histological picture of so-called primary healing of pressure osteosynthesis in experimental osteotomies in the dog. Experientia. 1963 Nov 15;19:593.

90. Schutze N, Kunzi-Rapp K, Wagemanns R, et al. 2005. Expression, purification, and functional testing of recombinant CYR61/CCN1. Protein Expr Purif 42:219–225.

91. Schutze N, Lechner A, Groll C, et al. 1998. The human analog of murine cystein rich protein 61 is a 1alpha,25-dihydroxyvitamin D3 responsive immediate early gene in human fetal osteoblasts: regulation

by cytokines, growth factors, and serum. Endocrinology 139:1761–1770.

92. Shah SB, Mishra AK, Chalise P, Shah RK, Singh RP, Shrivatava MP. Outcome of treatment of nonunion tibial shaft fracture by intramedullary interlocking nail augmentated with autogenous cancellous bone graft. Nepal Med Coll J. 2014 Sep;16(1):58-62

93. Tamura I, Rosenbloom J, Macarak E, et al. 2001. Regulation of Cyr61 gene expression by mechanical stretch through multiple signaling pathways. Am J Physiol Cell Physiol 281:C1524–C1532.

94. Thomas, T. A. The cell and molecular biology of fracture healing. Clinical Orthopaedics & Related Research.Fracture Healing Enhancement 1998; 1(355 Suppl), S7–S21.

95. Tonna, E. A. and Cronkite, E. P. Theperiosteum: autoradiographic studies on cellular proliferation and transformation utilizing tritiated thymidine. Clin.Orthop. 1963; 30, 218–233.

96. Virginie Fataccioli, Valérie Abergel, Laure Wingertsmann, Pascal Neuville, Estelle Spitz, Serge Adnot, Valérie Calenda, and Emmanuel Teiger. Stimulation of angiogenesis by Cyr61 gene: a new therapeutic candidate. Hum Gene Ther 2002;13: 1461–1470.

97. Weiliang Chua, Diarmuid Murphy, Weiming Siow, Fareed Kagda, Joseph Thambiah. Epidemiological analysis of outcomes in 323 open tibial diaphyseal fractures: a nine-year experience. Singapore Med J 2012; 53(6): 385–389

98. Wendeberg B. Mineral metabolism of fractures of the tibia in man studied with external counting of Sr85. Acta Orthopaedica Scandinavica. 1961 Dec 1;32(sup52):3-81.

99. Whelan DB, Bhandari M, Stephen D, Kreder H, McKee MD, Zdero R, Schemitsch EH. Development of the radiographic union scores for tibial fractures for the assessment of tibial fracture healing after intramedullary fixation. J Trauma. 2010; 68(3):629-32.

100. Wong M, Kireeva ML, Kolesnikova TV, et al. 1997. Cyr61, product of a growth factor-inducible immediate-early gene, regulates chondrogenesis in mouse limb bud mesenchymal cells. Dev Biol 192:492–508.

101. Yang GP, Lau LF. Cyr61, product of a growth factor-inducible immediate early gene, is associated with the extracellular matrix and the cell surface. Cell Growth Differ 1991;2:351–357.

www.ingramcontent.com/pod-product-compliance
Lightning Source LLC
Chambersburg PA
CBHW072000220326
41599CB00034BA/7072